Color Me Beautiful

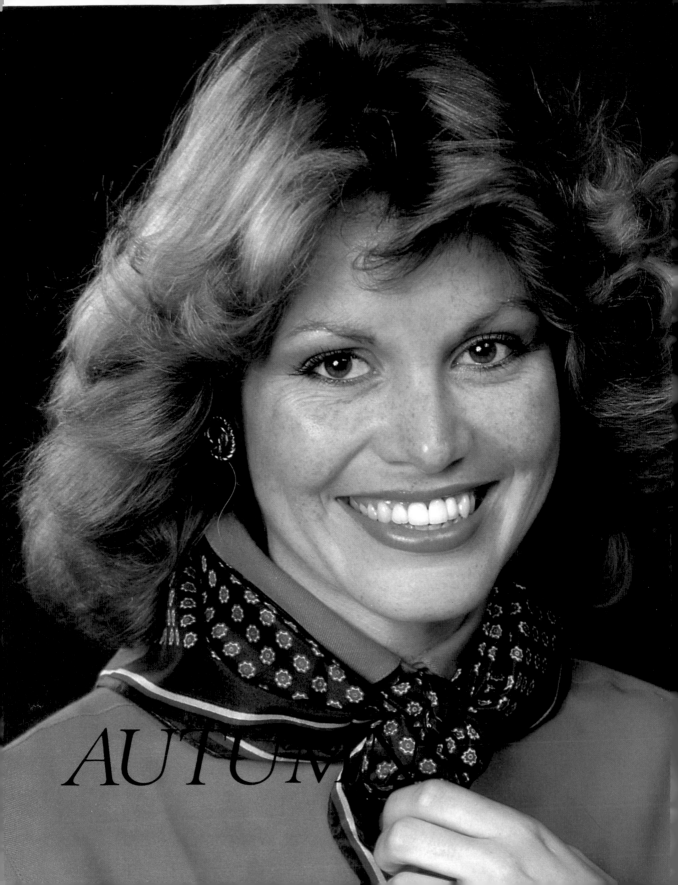
AUTUMN

Color Me Beautiful

Discover Your Natural Beauty Through The Colors That Make You Look Great & Feel Fabulous!

by Carole Jackson

Illustration by Christine Turner
Design by Robert Hickey
Makeup and Hair Styling by Susan Volk

BALLANTINE BOOKS · NEW YORK

For further information on clothing personality, see ART AND FASHION IN CLOTHING SELECTION by Harriet T. McJimsey, Second Edition © 1973 by the Iowa State University Press, Ames, Iowa 50010.

All models appearing in *Color Me Beautiful* were photographed by David Neely, Photo Concepts.

A special thanks to
Dorothy Douse and Frances Roller for appearing in *Color Me Beautiful*.

All other models in *Color Me Beautiful* are from The Model Store, Washington, D.C.

Katie Brown	Mary Heron	Kim Shanahan
Trena Brown	Pam Harris	Maura Shea
Margaret Connelly	Jennifer Klouman	Laurie Solow
Barbara Evans	Terri Moller	Susan Volk
Betsy Farley	Holly O'Dell	
Colleen Gaschen	Lisa Sanders	

Make-up and Hair Styling by Susan Volk

Library of Congress Catalog Card Number: 79-28456
ISBN 0-345-33294-6
This edition published by arrangement with Acropolis Books Ltd.

Manufactured in the United States of America
First Ballantine Books Edition: April 1981
Reprinted fifty-five times
Revised Ballantine Books Edition: September 1985

10 9 8 7 6 5 4 3

ACKNOWLEDGMENTS

This book has been fun to write. Everyone became involved, because color is contagious. People all along the chain of creating and promoting *Color Me Beautiful,* my publisher's staff, booksellers and book buyers from Maine to California, are now wearing their colors.

To those who gave their time and talent beyond the call of friendship or a paycheck, I give special thanks. First of all, to my associates in color, Mary Murphy and Sari Martin, who teach our classes in Scarsdale, New York. And then, for reasons they each know best, Winifred A. Adams, Cozy Baker, Bill B., Jeanne Brodsky, Andy Cella, Suzanne Greene, Kathleen Hughes, Margot Kline, Barbara Moore, Tom and Carla Nankervis, and Sandy Stewart. And especially, to John, for his thoughtful input, sensitivity, and friendship, and to Alec and Megan, for their enthusiasm and helpfulness from start to finish.

It is with equal gratitude that I acknowledge the women (and men) who have taken my classes and shared with me the joy of finding their colors.

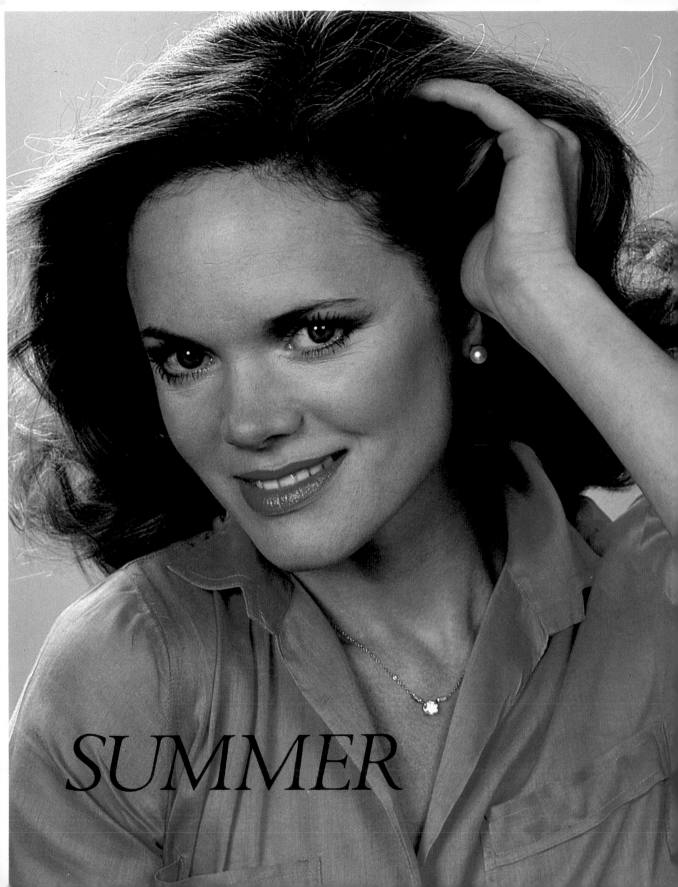

SUMMER

Color Me Beautiful

CONTENTS

SUMMER

WINTER

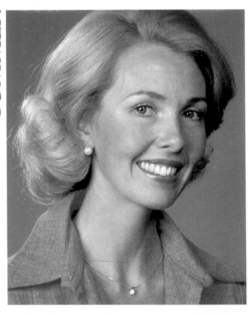

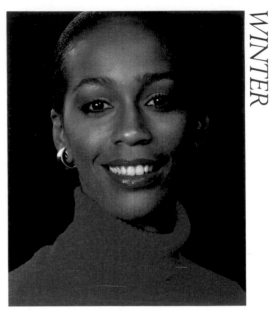

AUTUMN

SPRING

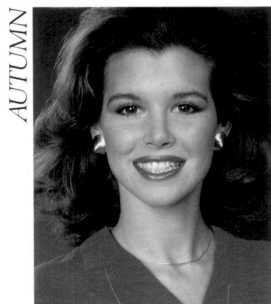

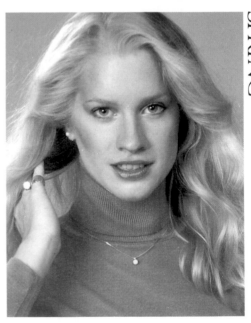

THE MAGIC OF COLOR

WHEN I WAS A YOUNG GIRL, I WANTED SO MUCH TO BE PRETTY. Studying myself in the mirror, I saw a pale, colorless face and decided that I really wasn't pretty at all. While the powder blue uniform required at my school made some of the girls look great, it did nothing for me. It in fact made me look gray, dull, and lifeless. The color of that daily uniform robbed me of some potentially good feelings about myself well into adult life.

Discovering lipstick and rouge as a teenager brought me instant life, but it was not until years later that I discovered the real magic of color. MY colors ... the missing link to finding my best self.

After having my coloring analyzed by a professional color consultant, I found that I do not look pale and lifeless after all—as long as I wear a color (the right blue, for example) that brings out the glow of my natural coloring. As I began wearing only the colors that were right for me, I started receiving compliments *all the time.* My colors had such an impact on my life that I wanted to share this exciting concept with others. You have special colors, too.

Each of us has a unique skin tone. Finding the colors that best complement this tone brings out our special beauty. I have seen many women literally come to life with radiance and new-found self-confidence as they discover their colors.

Perhaps you have never thought much about color, but I promise you that color has more impact than you ever imagined! Artists have studied its secrets and use them to make their masterpieces come alive. The world's most beautiful women—and men—have discovered its power to make the world regard them with awe.

Why do you picture Elizabeth Taylor in vivid, clear colors—royal blue, emerald green—and Candice Bergen in pastels? Why did your friend look fabulous on Monday, yet why did you walk right past her on Tuesday without saying hello because you didn't notice her? Why do you always reach for that certain dress in your own closet?

The answer is color.

Six years ago, after formal study of color and its application to clothing, makeup, and hair, I set up classes to teach women of all ages how to put themselves together from head to toe using their colors as the foundation. Over the years these classes have been refined, and they are the basis for this book.

At these "Color Me Beautiful" classes, we analyze each client's coloring, give her a packet of fabric swatches in her color palette, and teach her how to use them as a guide for shopping and looking beautiful. We spend one session on individual makeup, another on hair, one on personality and style, and one on wardrobe planning.

In our classrooms we use the seasons to describe people. For just as nature has divided herself into four distinct seasons, Autumn, Spring, Winter, and Summer, each with its unique and harmonious colors, your genes have given you a type of coloring that is most complemented by one of these seasonal palettes.

The Autumn is the woman who radiates in the warm, rich colors of fall, with their golden undertones, as crisp and colorful as the October leaves. The Spring woman blossoms in clear, delicate colors with warm yellow undertones, like the first daffodil that blooms each spring. The Winter woman sparkles in the vivid, clear primary colors, and cool, icy colors, like a glittering snowflake. And Summer glows in the pastels of June, the soft colors of the sea and sky, with their cool, blue undertones.

Through this book you will discover *your* season and learn which colors make you look fabulous all the time. After you know your best colors, you will move on to learn exactly what makeup and hair tones are perfect for you. Then we'll plan your wardrobe.

Color *is* magic and now let it work for you!

By the end of this book you will have color power—the ability to make the right fashion choices for yourself, to project your best image ... the power to be beautiful on the outside, to feel beautiful on the inside.

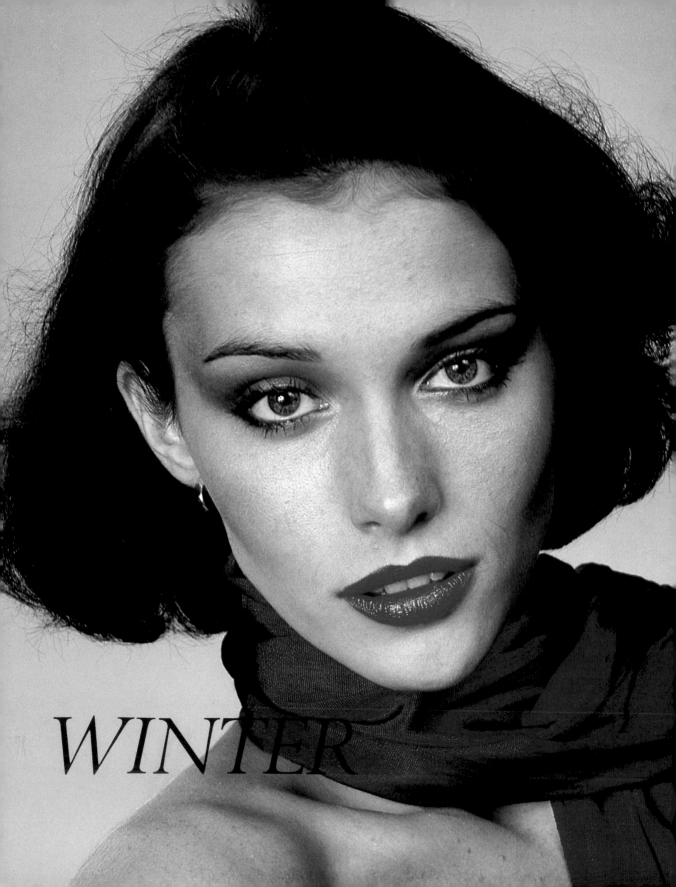

WINTER

Color Me Beautiful

I

Find Your Colors
Find Yourself

1

LET'S START WITH YOU

THE FIRST STEP IN FINDING THE COLORS THAT ARE PERFECT FOR you is a self-evaluation. Your answers to the following questions may help you increase your awareness of your clothes-buying and beauty habits. In addition, believe it or not, each question relates to color.

1. Can you wear *any* color and look terrific?

2. Do you create a good first impression *all the time?*

3. Do you have a closetful of clothes but nothing to wear?

4. Do you feel guilty about spending money on clothes?

5. Are you a compulsive clothes buyer?

6.   Are there any mistakes hanging in your closet?

7.   When you shop, do you have direction, or do you wander aimlessly through the store? Are you sure that everything you buy will be smashing and will blend with the rest of your wardrobe?

8.   Can you pack one suitcase for a two-week trip?

9.   Do you buy too much makeup, or no makeup at all, because you aren't sure what is just right for you?

10.   If you color your hair, are you positive that it is the most flattering shade?

11.   Are you excited about the way you look?

12.   Do you have "colorisma"?

If any *one* of your answers does not please you, *Color Me Beautiful* can help. By finding and learning to use your colors, you can achieve just what you want, whether it's a little change here and there, or an entirely new look. Then you can be happy with your answers to all these questions, for color—your personal palette—makes all the pieces fall into place. You'll look better; you'll shop more intelligently; and—if you're like the women who have taken my classes—you'll be excited about your looks and yourself.

The answer to the first question will always be "no." You need *your* colors to look terrific. Read on to find out why and how—then take the color test and discover your own season!

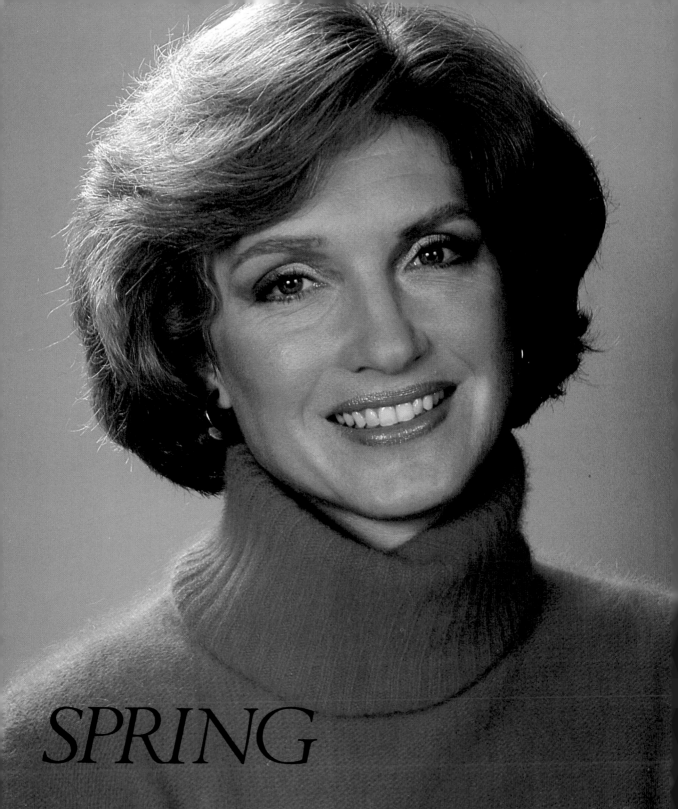

SPRING

2

COLOR MAKES THE DIFFERENCE

EVERYONE IS BORN WITH AN INCLINATION TOWARD CERTAIN colors. I have found that a very young child, before being influenced by parents and peers, will invariably pick out colors that suit her, sometimes to the horror of mother. One of my clients brought in her four-year-old for a color analysis. "Every time we go shopping she wants a black dress!" wailed the frustrated parent. The child was a Winter and black was indeed her color. Mom was a Spring, at home in camel and peach.

By the time we grow up, we may have lost a portion of that personal color sense, and we buy colors for reasons that don't have anything to do with how we look in them. We have been bombarded with color messages from mother (whose best colors may be different from our own) and from the fashion and home-furnishings industries, who use every medium available to popularize the colors they wish to sell.

Take heart. Nature usually prevails, and chances are good that at least 50 percent of your clothes are the right colors. And you probably already know which ones they are; they're the ones that make you feel great! Soon all your clothes will make you feel that way.

I was a bit skeptical when I had my colors analyzed years ago, but when I tried one of my new shades, the result was remarkable. I chose a royal blue turtleneck, a daring color for me, and wore it to a meeting one night when my mood was down. As I walked through the door, I received a compliment (a compliment to *me,* not my sweater). Dubious of this unexpected praise, I glanced in the mirror and discovered that I did indeed look better than I felt. My mood perked. By the end of the evening, after many compliments, I felt radiant and could hardly wait to try *all* my colors.

Today I wear only the colors of my seasonal palette because I feel attractive and confident in them. During my years as a color consultant, I have found that matching people with their colors produces immeasurable happiness.

Here are some real-life examples:

Jenny came to me in the middle of her diet. She had lost sixty pounds, had sixty more to go, and there was no stopping her. She was thrilled with her colors and had the pleasure of replacing her wardrobe quickly because she was rapidly growing too small for her clothes. Fortunately, she was developing self-esteem and was willing to buy attractive clothes even though she planned to be

Text continued on page 23.

WRONG COLOR

RIGHT COLOR

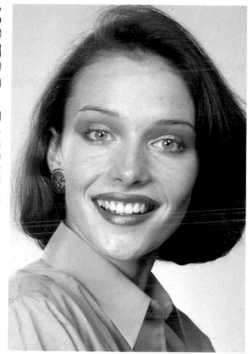
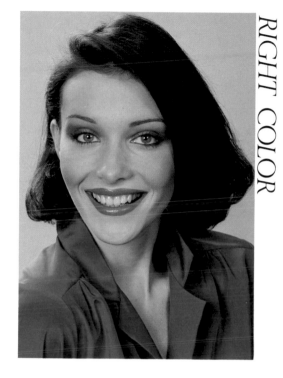

Margaret

Margaret *is a Winter with gray-blue eyes, dark ash brown hair and fair skin with a blue undertone. Her coloring is best complemented by clothes and makeup in cool, clear colors.*

In the picture on the left Margaret is wearing a gold shirt and orange-toned makeup. She looks pale and plain. But in the picture on the right, she is wearing royal blue with cool-toned makeup: a blue-red lipstick and pink blush . See how radiant she looks!

Color made the difference because both pictures were taken in the same studio, by the same photographer, using the same lighting.

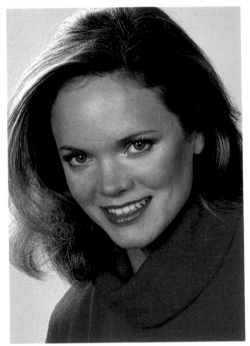

Mary

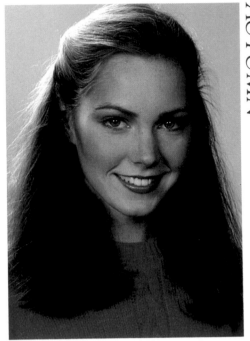

Kim

Mary *and* Kim *both have green eyes and brown hair, yet they are different seasons. Mary has a pink skin tone and looks best in cool colors with blue undertones, like the fuchsia she is wearing above. Kim's skin is ivory with golden highlights and she is most flattered by warm colors with yellow undertones, as in her orange sweater. Mary is a Summer; Kim is an Autumn. Notice that Mary's hair has a taupe (grayish) cast while Kim's hair has golden red highlights. Mary's green eyes have a hint of blue in them; Kim's have gold tones.*

Many green- or brown-eyed Summers mistakenly think they are Autumns. In the pictures at right Mary and Kim are wearing the same two turtlenecks, camel from the Autumn palette and pink from the Summer palette. Each changed her lipstick and blusher to go with the color of her shirt. See how Summer Mary looks drab in the yellow-tone camel and orange lipstick, but comes to life in the pink shirt and pink makeup tones that are so complementary to her natural coloring. By contrast, Kim is pale in the cool pink tones, but looks bright and healthy in the camel shirt and orange-tone makeup.

WRONG COLOR

RIGHT COLOR

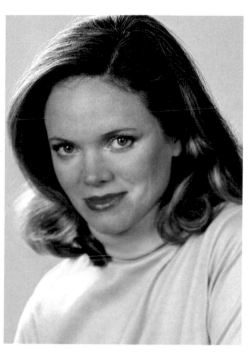
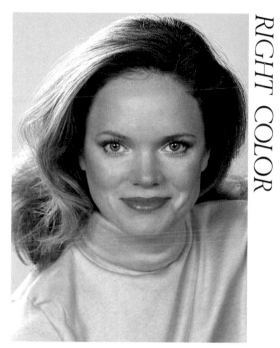

WRONG COLOR

RIGHT COLOR

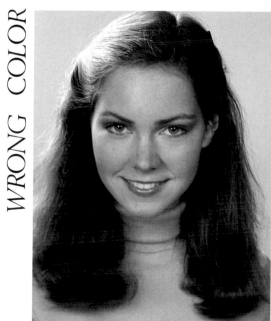
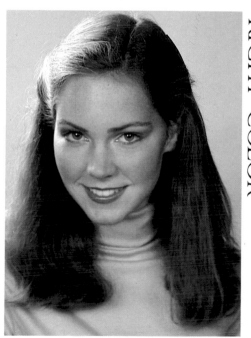

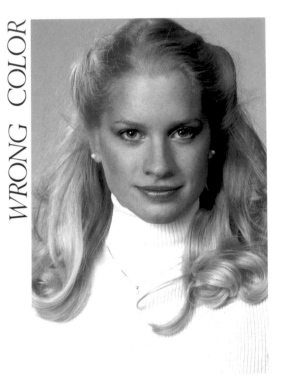

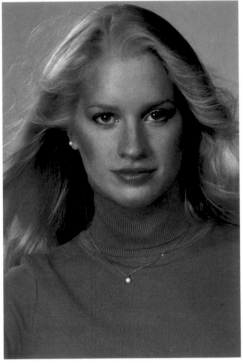

Susan

Susan, *a Spring, has an ivory skin tone, clear green eyes, and golden blonde hair. She looks best when she wears clear, yellow-toned colors. On the left she is wearing pure white, which drains the color from her face. But when she wears the coral pink sweater, in the picture on the right, her face comes to life—even in the same makeup.*

Susan's best white is ivory, a creamy white with a yellow undertone. Place a piece of ivory paper over her white sweater and see how much more flattering the ivory is.

A Winter is the only season who is truly flattered by pure white. Turn to page 27 to see Margaret, a Winter, in pure white. She would look pale in ivory.

Continued from page 18.

too small for them the next year (she was). My phone rang for months as Jenny's friends saw her transformation and wanted the same for themselves.

Pam was depressed. She had lost the ability to make even minor decisions and really had lost interest in life. A friend dragged her to my classes in hopes of cheering her up. She was obviously pleased with the rave reviews of the class as we draped her in her colors. But she was still afraid to go shopping. I finally gave her an assignment. She was to go to a department store and buy one blouse (which she said she needed). The next week, she came in beaming. "It was so easy," she said. "I didn't even look at half the things on the rack because they weren't my colors. I only took a few blouses into the dressing room and the second one I tried on looked so good that I didn't bother with the others. I bought it and here I am."

Marnie was a Summer whose hair had darkened. Her mother was an Autumn, and Marnie had spent her childhood in Autumn colors. Even now she wore mostly earth colors. She felt drab and wanted to do something to her hair, but she wasn't sure what. Draping her in Summer colors brought her to life. She was radiant. She frosted her hair just the right shade and looked stunning. Marnie also sells cosmetics and has found that her understanding of the seasonal palettes helps her tremendously with her clients.

"Help!" said Kathy. "I need a new image." Kathy was overweight and came to class in blue jeans, with her blonde hair in two ponytails. At age thirty-three, she obviously hadn't found herself. By the end of the six-week course, she had shed fifteen pounds, sported a chic, short haircut, and looked fabulous in her new makeup and a skirt and blouse in her colors. Six weeks later she had lost fifteen more pounds and had found a whole new identity. Kathy was one of my first students, and, six years later, I am happy to report that she is still skinny, looks great, and has obtained her credentials as a therapist.

Helen came to me right after her divorce. She had gone back to school, at age fifty, to prepare herself for reentry into the job market. Her colors, make-up, and a wardrobe plan for a working woman brought her up-to-date. She later wrote: "Getting my colors is the nicest thing I've done for myself in years. I felt so good on my job interviews, and I am sure my new boss thinks I'm ten years younger than I am!"

Marie was laughing when she came to the last class. "I went to my doctor and he wouldn't believe I wasn't feeling well because I look so good. He says I've never looked healthier in all the time he's known me." Marie was a pale Autumn who had never worn makeup. To camouflage the gray that was creeping into her hair, she had frosted it a silvery ash blonde—wrong for her. With her colors, a little blush and lipstick, and a change to auburn hair, she was indeed a new woman.

A few weeks after her color consultation, Charlotte wrote: "Such fantastic results! I never knew how great I could look. All I did was buy five new shirts in my more vivid colors. Although I wear them with the same skirts, there has been an instant change in my appearance. Suddenly I look alive and happy and *everyone* responds positively to the change. Even my clients have commented on my 'new' image.... I love the compliments. And I love the new me. Thanks for introducing me to myself!"

The discovery of color transformed each of these women. Color does make a difference—often a dramatic one. The fun is in the discovery; the rewards last a lifetime.

3

THE SEASONAL PALETTES

WINTER, SUMMER, SPRING, OR FALL—WHO'S THE FAIREST OF THEM all? You are!

Nature is the most brilliant designer of all, and the secret is in her seasons. Each season presents a distinct array of colors, and *your* coloring is in harmony with one of these palettes. We could call your coloring "Type A," "Type B," and so on, but comparison with the seasons provides a more aesthetic and poetic way to describe your coloring and your best colors.

Some women are their most beautiful in the clear, true primary colors or the icy colors of Winter, while others are flattered more by the softer shades of Summer. Autumns come to life in the rich, warm tones of fall, and the Spring woman's coloring is most enhanced by clear, warm colors, like the budding growth and fresh fruit tones of springtime. When you wear your special colors, you are indeed the fairest of them all.

The genes that determine your skin tone, hair, and eye color also determine what colors look best on you. When you study your coloring, you will find that your skin, hair, and eyes have either blue or golden tones. Your inherited skin tone does not change; it simply deepens with a tan and fades with age. The same colors will always look the best on you.

In our classes, we drape each client in all the colors of her season, contrasting wrong colors for the sake of comparison and illustration. The right color brings out the best, while the wrong shade detracts. It's exciting to see the differences. Many women do not know how pretty they are.

Before you take the color test, let's look carefully at the palettes. The Winter palette has either blue-based colors or true colors—colors with a balance between yellow and blue, black and white. The Summer colors have either blue, rose, or gray undertones. Because of these undertones, Winter and Summer are the *cool* palettes. Autumn's colors are based on golden tones, and Spring's have clear, yellow undertones. These are the *warm* palettes. Your coloring, like your palette, is either cool (blue) or warm (golden).

Study the characteristics of each seasonal palette, noting especially the differences in the beiges, blues, greens, pinks, and reds. Do you see, for example, that the Spring palette has clear yellow-greens, while Autumn has both yellow-greens and earth greens? Winter's greens are true or icy, and the Summer palette contains only blue-greens. Summers and Winters wear blue-reds (cool), while Springs and Autumns look best in orange-reds (warm). Spring's pinks have yellow in them; Summer's are blue-pinks; Winter's are true and vivid or icy; and Autumn has no pink.

Text continued on page 37.

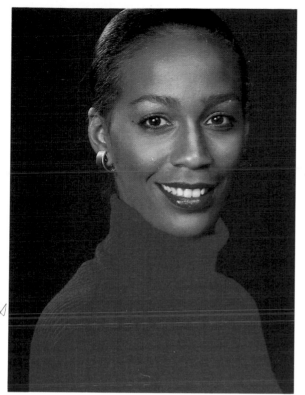

Trena

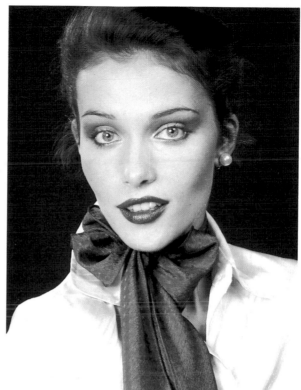

Margaret

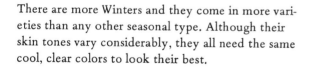

There are more Winters and they come in more varieties than any other seasonal type. Although their skin tones vary considerably, they all need the same cool, clear colors to look their best.

Trena is typical of many black Winters, with deep black-brown eyes, blue-black highlights in her hair, and a blue undertone to her skin.

Winters are the only ones who can wear black and pure white well. They come alive in true, vivid, and icy colors with a blue undertone. Note that Trena's sweater is a blue-red. There are no orange tones in the Winter palette.

Margaret is a typical Winter with her milky white skin, gray-blue eyes, and dark ash brown hair. Note that her hair's blue-black sheen has no red highlights, and her eyes have white flecks in the iris, characteristic of Winters.

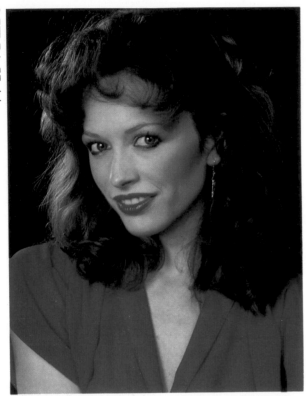

Betsy

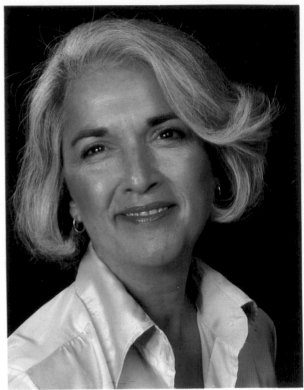

Frances

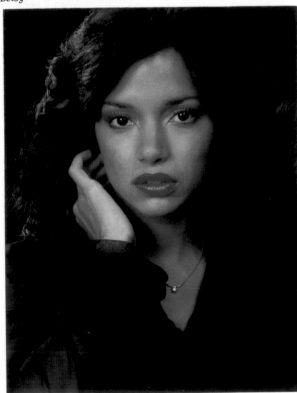

Pam

Betsy has a pink skin tone, blue eyes with dark gray rims around the iris, and brown hair. Although her hair picks up some red highlights from the sun, its basic tone is ash brown. Compare these highlights with the true, metallic red tones in the hair of Autumn Laurie on page 32.

Frances's hair began to turn from black-brown to a silvery gray in her early twenties. Prematurely gray hair is most typical of Winters, and Winters tend to gray attractively, as you can see. Frances's skin tone is deep rose-beige and her eyes are a rosy brown.

Dark-eyed, raven-haired **Pam** has olive skin. Although olive skin often appears golden, it actually has a blue undertone. Olive-skinned people and most blacks and Orientals look radiant in clear, vivid, cool colors, but sallow in warm colors. Most Winters have blue or brown eyes, but some have clear green, gray-green, or hazel eyes with a gray tone. Young Winters often have light brown hair, though it usually darkens with age.

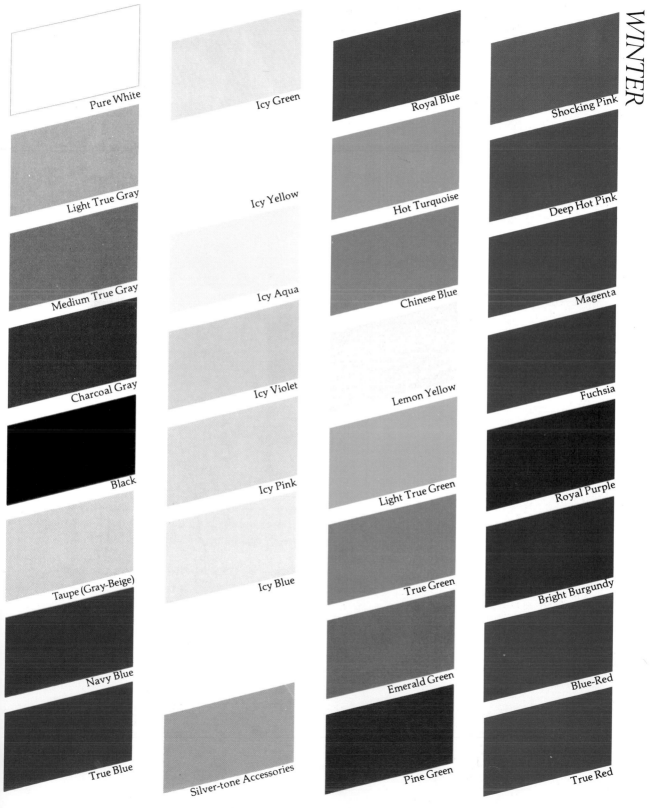

WINTER

Pure White

Light True Gray

Medium True Gray

Charcoal Gray

Black

Taupe (Gray-Beige)

Navy Blue

True Blue

Icy Green

Icy Yellow

Icy Aqua

Icy Violet

Icy Pink

Icy Blue

Silver-tone Accessories

Royal Blue

Hot Turquoise

Chinese Blue

Lemon Yellow

Light True Green

True Green

Emerald Green

Pine Green

Shocking Pink

Deep Hot Pink

Magenta

Fuchsia

Royal Purple

Bright Burgundy

Blue-Red

True Red

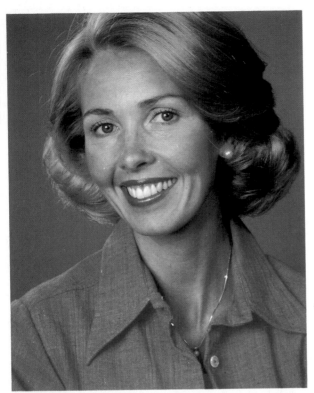

Terri

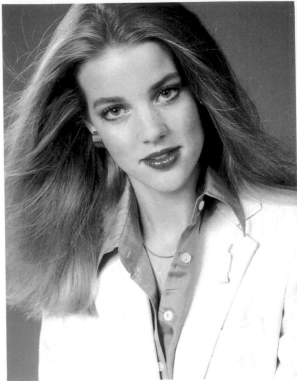

Katie

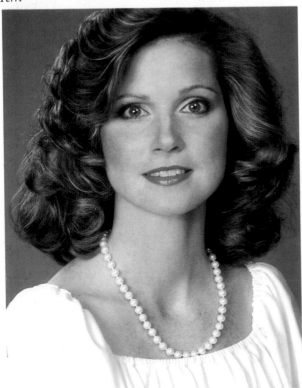

Barb

Terri is a typical Summer with her rosy pink skin tone, blue eyes, and ash blonde hair. To keep the blonde look, Terri highlights her hair with an ash blonde rinse.

Katie's fair skin is almost translucent with a blue undertone. Her aqua-gray eyes change from blue to green, depending on what she is wearing.

Barb is the freckled type. Her Summer eyes are deep blue with white flecks, and her hair is medium brown. Summer is the only season who can successfully frost her hair, because silver tones complement her blonde complexion.

Summer's eyes can also be green, hazel, or occasionally rosy brown. Most Summers have blonde, light brunette, or dark ash brown hair. The Summer is flattered by soft colors with a blue undertone. Note Barb's dress is a soft white (not ivory), and Terri's blouse is a blue-pink rather than the coral pink worn by Susan, a Spring, on page 22.

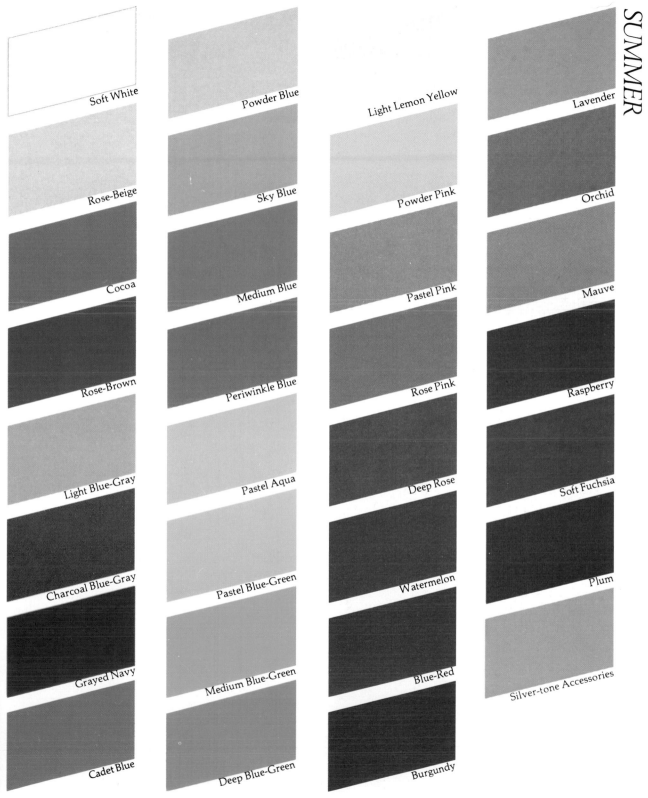

SUMMER

Soft White
Rose-Beige
Cocoa
Rose-Brown
Light Blue-Gray
Charcoal Blue-Gray
Grayed Navy
Cadet Blue

Powder Blue
Sky Blue
Medium Blue
Periwinkle Blue
Pastel Aqua
Pastel Blue-Green
Medium Blue-Green
Deep Blue-Green

Light Lemon Yellow
Powder Pink
Pastel Pink
Rose Pink
Deep Rose
Watermelon
Blue-Red
Burgundy

Lavender
Orchid
Mauve
Raspberry
Soft Fuchsia
Plum
Silver-tone Accessories

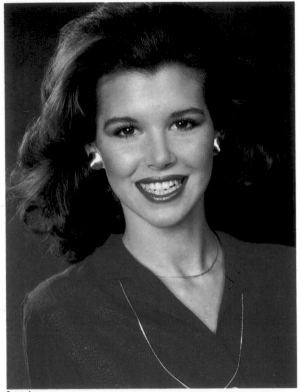

Laurie

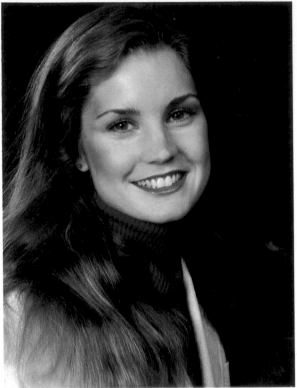

Maura

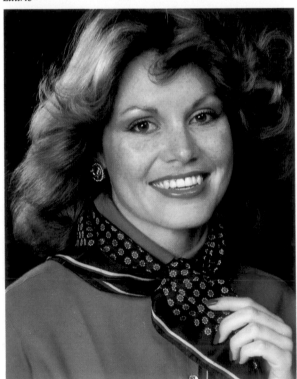

Colleen

Laurie is a vivid Autumn with fiery red highlights in her hair and dark golden brown eyes.

Maura's skin tone is ivory, and she is especially flattered by the muted Autumn tones, such as the bittersweet red turtleneck she is wearing under her oyster white jacket. Note the golden green color of Maura's eyes and her golden brown hair, typical of the Autumn.

Colleen has a true peach skin tone underneath those freckles. Her avocado green eyes and golden blonde hair make her an Autumn. Only an Autumn can look this terrific in pumpkin and olive green.

Most Autumns have brown, green, or hazel eyes, but a few have bright turquoise eyes (usually the redheads). Autumn hair invariably has gold or red highlights, whether blonde, brunette, or vivid redhead. Carrot-tops are usually Autumns.

The Autumn is complemented by warm colors with golden undertones. Note that Laurie's lipstick is brick red and her blouse is an orange-red rather than the blue-red worn by Trena on page 27.

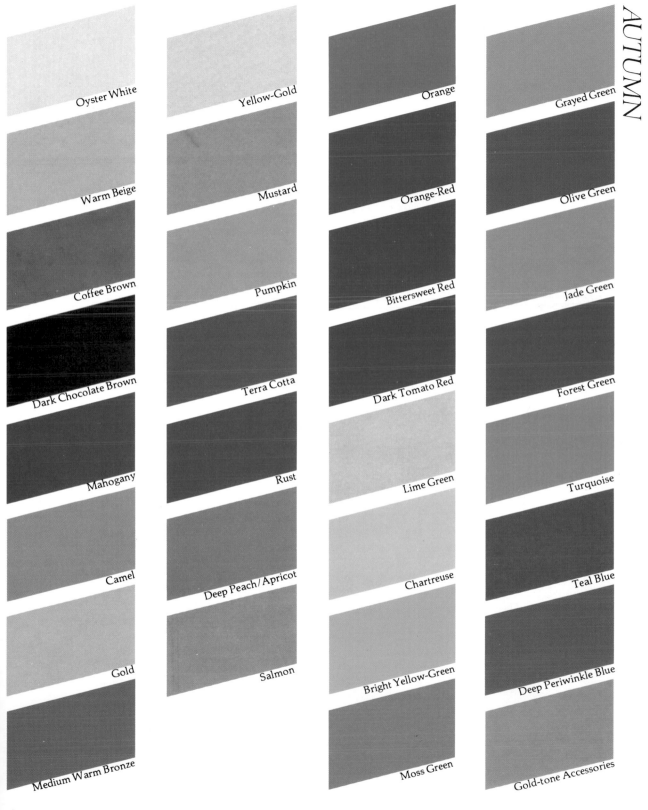

AUTUMN

Oyster White

Warm Beige

Coffee Brown

Dark Chocolate Brown

Mahogany

Camel

Gold

Medium Warm Bronze

Yellow-Gold

Mustard

Pumpkin

Terra Cotta

Rust

Deep Peach/Apricot

Salmon

Orange

Orange-Red

Bittersweet Red

Dark Tomato Red

Lime Green

Chartreuse

Bright Yellow-Green

Moss Green

Grayed Green

Olive Green

Jade Green

Forest Green

Turquoise

Teal Blue

Deep Periwinkle Blue

Gold-tone Accessories

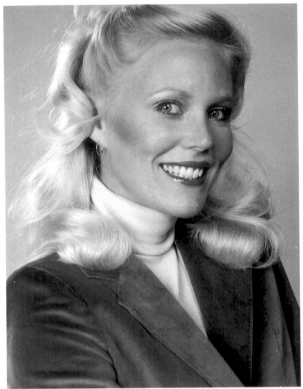

Holly

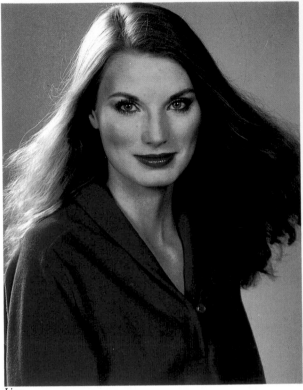

Lisa

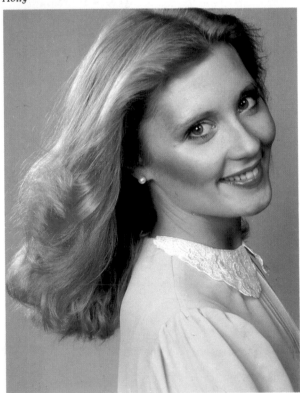

Jennifer

Holly is a typical Spring with her golden blonde hair, blue-green eyes, and peachy skin tone.

Lisa is a Spring with vivid red hair, and she looks especially good in her palette's brightest colors. Her fair ivory skin and pale blue eyes have a delicate quality, characteristic of many Springs.

Jennifer's ivory complexion looks like peaches and cream and is most flattered by Spring's softer colors, like the peach she is wearing. Her auburn hair is characteristic of Spring, as are her deep blue eyes with their pale yellow flecks.

Though many Springs are blonde in childhood, their hair usually darkens with age, retaining its golden cast. Flaxen blondes, like Holly and Susan on page 22, are the lucky ones who stay blonde naturally. Springs can have blue, green, hazel, or amber eyes, usually with golden tones. Notice that Spring Dorothy, on page 16, has blue eyes with a turquoise cast.

The Spring palette contains clear, warm colors, some delicate, some bright—all with yellow undertones. Note Holly's golden brown jacket. A darker brown is too harsh for her coloring.

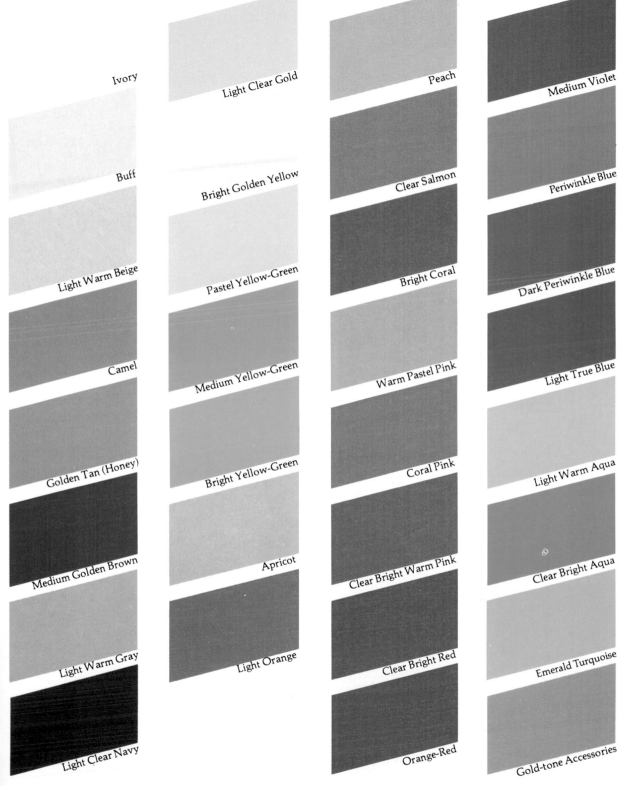

SPRING

Ivory

Buff

Light Warm Beige

Camel

Golden Tan (Honey)

Medium Golden Brown

Light Warm Gray

Light Clear Navy

Light Clear Gold

Bright Golden Yellow

Pastel Yellow-Green

Medium Yellow-Green

Bright Yellow-Green

Apricot

Light Orange

Peach

Clear Salmon

Bright Coral

Warm Pastel Pink

Coral Pink

Clear Bright Warm Pink

Clear Bright Red

Orange-Red

Medium Violet

Periwinkle Blue

Dark Periwinkle Blue

Light True Blue

Light Warm Aqua

Clear Bright Aqua

Emerald Turquoise

Gold-tone Accessories

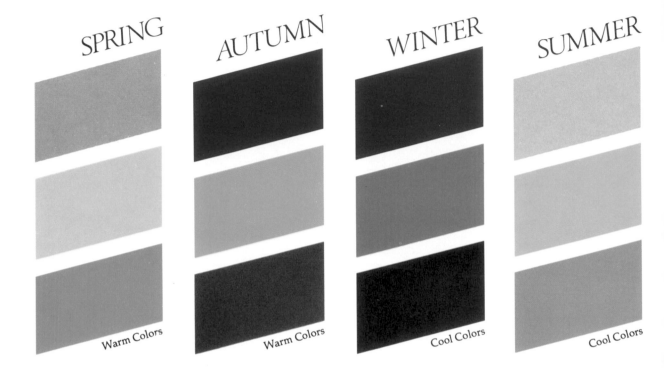

SPRING

AUTUMN

WINTER

SUMMER

Warm Colors

Warm Colors

Cool Colors

Cool Colors

You can wear almost any color; it's the shade and intensity that count. Spring's colors are clear, delicate, or bright with yellow undertones. Autumn's colors are stronger with orange and gold undertones. Winter's colors are clear, vivid, or icy with blue undertones. And Summer's colors are cool and soft with blue undertones.

Continued from page 26

Now examine the palettes for intensity. Although Winter and Summer are both cool, the depth of their colors varies considerably. The same is true of Autumn's and Spring's warm palettes. Winter's colors are all clear, true, vivid, or icy, while Summer's colors may be either clear or powdered (muted) and are always less intense. While Winter has royal purple, Summer has plum, a muted purple. Note the differences in the intensity of the blues, pinks, greens, and yellows. Note, too, the differences in the Winter and Summer models. Winter coloring is stronger, with greater contrast in skin, hair, and eyes. Summer has softer, less intense coloring. The warm Autumn palette is strong, with both vivid and muted colors. But Spring has only *clear* colors, either bright or delicate, but never muted or extremely dark. Notice the differences in the golds, browns, greens, beiges, and oranges of these two seasons. See how much darker the Autumn models' hair and eyes are compared to the delicate coloring of the Spring models.

A few colors are missing entirely from some of the palettes, and other colors are unique to just one palette. Winter is the only season to have black and pure white. But Winter has no brown or orange. Autumn alone has very dark brown, but no navy, pink, or gray. Summer has no orange, and Spring has a little bit of every color except black and pure white.

In looking at the palettes, you may feel that you can wear colors from all the seasons. True, it is possible to find a few colors from each that might look good on you. Some colors are relatively flattering to everyone, which is nice if you need to outfit a quartet or a bevy of bridesmaids. Everyone can wear Summer's soft white (this is not a yellow-white). Other good colors for a group are Spring's corals and her light warm aqua, Autumn's deep periwinkle blue, and Summer's watermelon. These colors are not included in all the palettes, however, because they are a compromise for some.

There are two important reasons for *not* mixing palettes or "borrowing" colors from a palette that is not yours. First, you will look *best* in your own.

Why look good when it's just as easy to look great? Second, each palette has been carefully arranged to give you a well-coordinated wardrobe, consisting of compatible tones. If you buy colors helter-skelter, you will end up with a closetful of clothes and nothing to wear. As you build your wardrobe from the palette of your season, you will quickly benefit from this bonus. Because your colors go with each other, your outfits and accessories will coordinate all by themselves.

Perhaps you fear being restricted or bored wearing only one set of colors. But look at the variety in each season! Once into your palette, you will find instead that you have more colors to wear than you currently allow yourself— perhaps colors you never thought of trying. The truth is that you can wear almost any *color;* it's the *shade and intensity* that count! We are going to enrich and enlarge your wardrobe possibilities to some thirty shades that all look good on you. You won't be bored by your colors, and it's never boring to be beautiful.

The palettes are all designed to give you a wide range of colors, with something appropriate for every time of year and for every kind of occasion. Some of your colors are suitable for wintertime, some for summertime. Your palette contains sporty colors, dressy colors, neutrals, basics, and bright accent colors. You will find a color to suit your every mood and need.

The seasonal color theory was inspired by the studies of artist and colorist Johannes Itten of the famous Bauhaus school in Germany. He discovered the power of physical coloring in directing a student's choice of colors in his paintings. He noted that a student's personal colors were consistently those complementary to his skin tone, hair, and eyes, in both tone and intensity. After years of observation and documentation, he emphatically states in his book, *The Elements of Color* (page 27), that "Every woman should know what colors are becoming to her; these will always be her subjective colors and their complements. ..." So Itten concluded that our personal palette, the one to which we are drawn naturally, consists of the very colors that look best on us.

In adapting Itten's theory to fashion we have developed the four seasonal palettes as guides for clothing, makeup, and wardrobe planning. You don't have to be a brilliant colorist or fashion coordinator yourself, though you will look as if you are. Simply determine which palette fits your coloring, wear those colors, and enjoy the compliments.

Perhaps the biggest joy in finding your personal colors is the freedom it brings. Using your colors, you will spend less time and energy shopping, yet you will have more confidence than ever that you look your best. Shopping will become quick and easy, because you will know what to look for and what to leave on the racks. You won't waste money or clutter up your closet with mistakes. Your palette can be a tool that will simplify one aspect of your life, leaving you free to pursue other interests. It works for me. It works for others. It will work for you.

Now that you have been introduced to the palettes, let's go on to find your colors.

4

DETERMINING YOUR COLORS: The Color Test

NOW COMES THE FUN—FINDING *YOUR* COLORS! WITH THESE colors you can build a completely coordinated wardrobe, choose the right makeup, and create a new image that will truly reflect you.

The first step is to select key colors you have consistently worn with success throughout your lifetime. The second step is to evaluate your coloring—your skin, hair, and eyes. These two steps will tell you your season.

I am including a third optional step for those of you who would like to observe yourself in test colors, including makeup, the way we do in our classroom. This is best done in a group because it is difficult for people to see themselves objectively and other opinions are helpful. If you are already in a classroom situation, or perhaps a club, I strongly urge you to do Step 3 for the fun of it. It requires some effort to gather test colors, but the visual impact of seeing yourself and others in colors is most convincing!

STEP 1: YOUR COLOR HISTORY

Select the group of colors below which you feel is most flattering to you, in general. As Johannes Itten proved with his art students, you will intuitively know whether you are better in cool or warm colors. The Summer and Winter palettes contain cool, blue-based colors; Autumn and Spring contain warm, yellow-based colors. Do not base your decision on the clothes currently hanging in your closet. They may be right, but they may instead be the result of a current fad that is not necessarily for you! Pick the group containing the most colors that have brought you compliments all your life (even though you may be tired of wearing them). This test is based on comparison. Each column may have some colors that you have worn, but do they all look equally good on you? Ask yourself, "Which group is *best*?"

Cool		Warm	
WINTER	*SUMMER*	*AUTUMN*	*SPRING*
Navy	Soft Blues	Dark Brown	Golden Brown
Black	Rose-Brown	Camel	Camel
White	Navy	Beige	Peachy Pink
Red	Rose Pink	Orange	Peach
Shocking Pink	Lavender	Gold	Bright Blues
Gray	Plum	Moss Green	Golden Yellow

Now look at the printed palette of your choice, as well as the charts on pages 66 through 69. Does the whole palette seem to suit you? If so, go on to Step 2. If not, make a second choice from the color groups above, and then look at the palette for that season. If you are deciding between two seasons, ask yourself the following questions:

If you are deciding between

Winter and Autumn, ask:

Am I better in navy, pure white, and clear colors (Winter) or brown, pumpkin, and muted gold (Autumn)? Be careful. Some brown-eyed Winters think they're Autumns. Brown is boring on a Winter, exciting on an Autumn. Ask your friends.

Winter and Summer, ask:

Do I look good in pastels, like powder pink or blue (Summer), or do I need darker or brighter colors because pastels make me look washed out (Winter)?

Winter and Spring, ask:

Am I really terrific in ivory, camel, and golden browns (Spring) or am I better in navy, pure white, and dark colors (Winter)?

Summer and Autumn, ask:

Am I great in pastel blues and pinks but not good in pumpkin or mustard colors (Summer) or is it the other way around (Autumn)?

Summer and Spring, ask:

Which do I wear better, buff, yellow-green, peachy pinks, golden browns (Spring) or blue-greens, blue-pinks, burgundy, or rose-tone browns (Summer)?

Spring and Autumn, ask: Can I wear muted colors like mustard and moss green or very dark brown (Autumn) or am I better in clear colors like buff, light clear gold, peach, and lighter golden browns (Spring)? If neither seems quite right, try Summer. Many brown-eyed or green-eyed Summers mistakenly think they are warm seasons because they like camel, brown, and some greens. Summer has rose-brown, rose-beige, and many shades of blue-green.

Now pick your preferred season and move on to step 2.

STEP 2: A LOOK AT YOUR COLORING – THE SKIN TONE TEST

This step is to verify your selection in Step 1.

Take a long look at yourself in the mirror, near natural daylight if possible. Look at your skin, hair, and eyes, without makeup. If you color your hair, try to remember its natural color.

Your skin tone is the most important factor in determining the colors that look best on you. The tone of your skin comes from three pigments, melanin (brown), carotene (yellow), and hemoglobin (red). It is the particular combination of these three pigments that gives you your unique skin tone. Because your skin acts as a thin filter, it is the tone just under its surface that determines whether your coloring is cool or warm. Summers and Winters, the cool seasons, have blue undertones, while Autumns and Springs have golden undertones. Some people's skin tone is quite obvious, but for others the tone is subtle. In class, we compare wrists and palms. By comparison, you can often see whether you are more blue or golden than someone else. Take a piece of very white paper and hold it under your wrist and hand for comparison. Are you blue (or blue-pink) or are you golden (even orange)? If you have freckles, are they charcoal brown (cool) or golden brown (warm)?

Warning: Be careful not to confuse sallowness with a golden skin tone. Anyone can have sallow skin, which appears yellow on the surface, regardless of its undertone. By the same token, any season can have a ruddy complexion, where the capillaries are close to the surface of the skin, giving an intense pinkness to the face. This should not necessarily be confused with a blue tone, as, ironically, ruddiness occurs most often in the warm seasons.

If you are uncertain of your skin tone, or if you are sallow or ruddy, look in the mirror at your entire body, nude, especially the untanned portions. Again, comparison is helpful. For example, my olive skin appears yellow at first glance, but in comparison to my daughter's ivory body, I look "blue" and she looks "golden." She is an Autumn, I am a Winter.

Because your skin tone is not always obvious, here are more complete descriptions of the various types of coloring that typify each season, including hair and eyes. Read *only* the description of the season you selected in Step 1 and see if you find yourself. If you don't, then read the description of your second choice in Step 1. Combining your answers to Steps 1 and 2, pick whichever of these seasons you feel most suits you.

WINTER

Skin: First look for the blue or blue-pink undertone, but don't be discouraged if you can't readily see it. It's often subtle on a Winter. There are more Winters in the world than any other seasonal type. Winters may vary a great deal, yet they all need the same cool colors to look their best. The largest range of Winters in the United States are those with gray-beige skin, ranging from light to dark, usually with no visible pink in the skin. Most olive-skinned people, blacks, and Orientals are Winters, although a few are Summers, Autumns, or Springs. Many Winters are sallow, appearing yellow, and they misdiagnose themselves as Autumns. But golden colors will make them appear more sallow, while the cool Winter colors make their sallowness disappear. A Winter may also have milky white skin and dark hair (like Snow White). The white may have a visible pink tone or may appear pure white with a translucent quality. Winters do not usually have rosy cheeks, and their appearance improves dramatically with pink tone blusher.

Hair: Most Winters have dark hair, even though some were white-blonde in infancy. Brunette Winters have hair color ranging from light brown to dark charcoal brown. Winter's hair usually has an ash tone, although sometimes the hair will have a touch of red highlights visible in the sun. (Don't confuse this with the metallic red seen in Autumn's hair, however.) Blue-black hair is typical of Winter, as is salt-and-pepper or silver gray. It is common for a Winter to gray prematurely, and she often grays attractively. Rarely do we find a Winter who is naturally blonde as an adult, but if she is, her hair is white-blonde, giving her a striking look.

Eyes: The Winter woman's eyes are most often a deep color. They may be red-brown, black-brown, green, blue, hazel, gray-blue, gray-green, or dark blue. The blue- or green-eyed Winter has white flecks in the iris and often a gray rim around the edge of the iris. The hazel-eyed Winter usually has a brown smudge with jagged edges surrounding the pupil, with either blue or green extending to the outer iris. Occasionally, a green-eyed Winter has a thick yellow "line" going from the pupil to the outer edge of the iris like a single spoke on a wheel. In general, Winter eyes tend to have a look of high contrast between the whites of the eye and the iris. This clue is especially helpful if you are deciding between Winter and Summer, as the white of a Summer eye is usually much softer with less contrast to the iris.

Well-known Winters: Elizabeth Taylor, Cher, Jacqueline Onassis, Audrey Hepburn, Jaclyn Smith, Marie Osmond, Princess Caroline, Sally Field, Diana Ross.

WINTER

Check whichever characteristics describe you:

Skin:
- ☐ Very white
- ☐ White with delicate pink tone
- ☐ Beige (no cheek color, may be sallow)
- ☐ Gray-beige or brown
- ☐ Rosy beige
- ☐ Olive
- ☐ Black (blue undertone)
- ☐ Black (sallow)

Hair:
- ☐ Blue-black
- ☐ Dark brown (may have red highlights)
- ☐ Medium ash brown
- ☐ Salt-and-pepper
- ☐ Silver-gray
- ☐ White blonde (rare)
- ☐ White

Eyes:
- ☐ Dark red-brown
- ☐ Black-brown
- ☐ Hazel (brown plus green or blue)
- ☐ Gray-blue
- ☐ Blue with white flecks in iris (may have gray rim)
- ☐ Dark blue, violet
- ☐ Gray-green
- ☐ Green with white flecks in iris (may have gray rim)

SUMMER

Skin: Look for the blue undertone. Summers usually have visible pink in their skin. Some Summers are very fair and look pale without a little blush. These fair Summers may have a translucent quality to the skin with little pink rings showing under the skin on the whitest parts of the body; they are usually blonde, or were blonde in early childhood, and have light brown hair as they mature. Some Summers have very pink skin, with high color, while others have rose-beige skin, ranging from fair to relatively deep rose-beige. Other Summers have sallow beige skin, making it hard to see the blue undertone. Sallow Summers improve their appearance dramatically with Summer's cool colors. Black Summers have a soft grayish tone to their skin and their skin is fairly light. If you are deciding between Autumn and Summer, Summers usually tan while Autumns more often burn.

Hair: As a child, Summer is most often blonde, ranging from towhead to ash blonde to dark ash. As she matures, her hair tends to darken to a "mousy" color, so named because of its grayish cast. Brunette Summers also have hair color ranging from light to dark brown, again with ash overtones. Often a very dark-haired Summer has extremely light skin, and visible pink in her cheeks. Summer blondes bleach quickly in the sun, resulting in brownish hair in the wintertime and blonder hair in the summertime. Occasionally a Summer has warm blonde hair or hair with auburn highlights, especially if she gets lots of sun. This type of Summer can be mistaken for a Spring or Autumn. (Look at your roots to judge your hair color accurately.) The Summer woman grays gracefully (often prematurely) to a soft blue-gray or pearly white tone. Summers, of all the seasons, most often feel the need to "brighten" themselves with hair color or frosting. A Summer woman truly benefits from wearing her colors, as her colors alone bring "life" to her face.

Eyes: Summer eyes are most often blue, green, aqua, gray, or soft hazel (predominantly blue or green with grayed brown surrounding the pupil). The Summer eye often has a cloudy look inside the iris, rather than a clear, transparent color. The iris in a blue or green eye has a white webbing throughout, giving the appearance of cracked glass. Many Summers have soft gray eyes or eyes with a gray rim around the iris. Intensely blue eyes are characteristic of some lucky Summers, while other Summers have soft rose-brown or grayed brown eyes. The whites of a Summer's eyes are creamy, in soft contrast to the iris, as opposed to a Winter, whose eyes have sharp contrast.

Well-known Summers: Princess Grace of Monaco, Queen Elizabeth, Candice Bergen, Cheryl Tiegs, Farrah Fawcett, Nancy Kissinger, Caroline Kennedy.

SUMMER

Check whichever characteristics describe you:

Skin:

- ☑ Pale beige with delicate pink cheeks
- ☐ Pale beige with no cheek color (even sallow)
- ☐ Rosy beige
- ☐ Very pink
- ☐ Gray-brown
- ☐ Rosy brown

Hair:

- ☐ Platinum blonde
- ☐ Ash blonde (often towhead as a child)
- ☐ Warm ash blonde (slightly golden)
- ☐ Dark ash ("mouse") blonde
- ☐ Ash ("mouse") brown
- ☑ Dark brown (taupe tone)
- ☐ Brown with auburn cast
- ☐ Blue-gray
- ☐ Pearl white

Eyes:

- ☐ Blue (with white webbing in the iris, cloudy look)
- ☑ Green (with white webbing in the iris, cloudy look)
- ☐ Soft gray-blue
- ☐ Soft gray-green
- ☐ Bright, clear blue
- ☐ Pale, clear aqua (eyes change from blue to green, depending on clothes)
- ☐ Hazel (cloudy brown smudge with blue or green)
- ☐ Pale gray
- ☐ Soft rose-brown
- ☐ Grayed brown

AUTUMN

Skin: Look for the golden undertone. The Autumn comes in three varieties: the fair person with ivory or creamy peach skin; the true redhead, fair to dark, often with freckles; and the golden-beige brunette, whose skin ranges from medium to deep copper, the latter having charcoal black hair. Many Autumns are pale or sallow and especially need an orange-tone rouge to "come alive." An Autumn and a Spring may have similar coloring, but the Autumn will usually have colorless cheeks, while Spring's cheeks will be rosy. Some Autumns are ruddy, however, and may look pink, but the pink is more peachy than blue. These Autumns look good in a few Summer colors, but really come to life in the true Autumn palette. A few Orientals and blacks are Autumns, if they have a truly golden undertone, but most are other seasons.

Hair: Autumn can be golden blonde as a child, usually darkening as she matures. Autumn's hair is most often touched with red or golden highlights. It ranges from auburn to copper, strawberry blonde to carrot top, dark golden blonde to warm brown. (A few redheads are Springs, having coloring too delicate to handle the stronger Autumn palette.) Many Autumns are brunette, their hair usually having a gold or metallic red cast. Some Autumns have ash blonde hair that has no warm highlights. This type of "dirty" blonde Autumn can be easily confused with a Summer. Occasionally, an Autumn has charcoal black hair and swarthy skin. A red-headed Autumn should cover gray, as it tends to come in yellow-gray, and the two-tone look is drab on her. However, once her hair is completely gray, it can be most attractive.

Eyes: Most Autumns have golden brown eyes, from dark to topaz, or green eyes with orange or golden streaks radiating from a star formation that surrounds the pupil. Isolated flecks, either gold, brown, or black, are often present in the Autumn eye. Some Autumns have clear green eyes, like glass, or deep olive green "cat" eyes. An Autumn's hazel eye contains golden brown, green, and gold. A few Autumns have vivid turquoise, aqua, or steel blue eyes that are marked by a teal gray rim around the edge of the iris. Occasionally, an Autumn has extremely pale blue or teal eyes, giving the appearance of a clear ring around the pupil. This is a pastel Autumn who looks best in the muted colors of the palette.

Well-known Autumns: Vanessa Redgrave, Carol Burnett. Shirley MacLaine, Ann-Margret, Toni Tenille, Katharine Hepburn, Lucille Ball, Maggie Smith.

AUTUMN

Check whichever characteristics describe you:

Skin:

- ☐ Ivory
- ☐ Ivory with freckles (usually redhead)
- ☐ Peach
- ☐ Peach with freckles (usually golden blonde, brown)
- ☐ Golden beige (no cheek color, needs blush)
- ☐ Dark beige (coppery)
- ☐ Golden brown

Hair:

- ☐ Red
- ☐ Coppery red-brown
- ☐ Auburn
- ☐ Golden brown (dark honey)
- ☐ Golden blonde (honey)
- ☐ Ash ("dirty") blonde
- ☐ Strawberry blonde
- ☐ Charcoal brown or black
- ☐ Golden gray
- ☐ Oyster white

Eyes:

- ☐ Dark brown
- ☐ Golden brown
- ☐ Amber
- ☐ Hazel (golden brown, green gold)
- ☐ Green (with brown or gold flecks)
- ☐ Pale, clear green
- ☐ Olive green
- ☐ Blue with a distinct aqua or turquoise tone
- ☐ Teal blue
- ☐ Steel blue

SPRING

Skin: Look for the golden undertone. Springs have the most delicate quality of all the seasonal types. Spring's skin is either creamy ivory, peachy pink, peach, or golden beige. Freckles come naturally to her, though some Springs have skin clear as glass, often called "peaches and cream." The ivory Spring appears to have golden flecks or highlights to her skin, while the peachy Spring is likely to have peachy pink cheeks. Of all the seasons, Springs are the most likely to have rosy cheeks and to flush easily. Their skin is usually finely textured, and color seems to rush to the surface. Some Springs are very ruddy and can be confused with Summers because of the apparent pinkness. Even their knuckles look purple. Look at the parts of your body that don't blush to see whether you are peach or truly pink. Springs have an aliveness and brightness to their skin tone, even if they are extremely fair. Black and Oriental Springs have light, golden brown skin.

Hair: Spring's hair is flaxen blonde, yellow blonde, honey, strawberry, taffy-red, or golden brown. Ash-tone hair is not Spring. In childhood many Springs are blonde, ranging from flaxen to honey to strawberry, but their hair often darkens with age. Some have very dark brown hair. A few Springs are vivid carrot-tops, missing being Autumns by their need for clear colors. Gray does not blend with the golden hair of a Spring, so she is wise to keep her hair dyed its youthful color until she has turned totally gray. Once the two-tone look is gone, her gray hair is a beautiful creamy white or a pale, dove gray.

Eyes: Spring's eyes are likely to be blue, green, teal, or aqua often with golden flecks in the iris or a golden cluster around the pupil. Some Springs have eyes as clear as glass, giving the impression of a clear ring around the pupil. Many Springs have blue eyes that appear to be a solid steel gray from a distance, but up close, they are really blue and have a sunburst of white "rays" coming from the pupil. Inside the sunburst you may see a doughnut tightly surrounding the pupil. Fibers radiate from the edge of the sunburst to the edge of the iris, much like the spokes of a wheel. There are some brown-eyed Springs, but they are always golden brown or topaz. A Spring's hazel eye contains golden brown, green, and gold.

Well-known Springs: Sally Struthers, Joan Kennedy, Zsa Zsa and Eva Gabor, Debbie Reynolds, Shirley Jones, Julie Andrews, Arlene Dahl, Marilyn Monroe.

SPRING

Check whichever characteristics describe you:

Skin:
- ☐ Creamy ivory
- ☐ Ivory with pale golden freckles
- ☐ Peach
- ☐ Peach/pink (may have pink/purple knuckles)
- ☐ Golden beige
- ☐ Rosy cheeks (may blush easily)
- ☐ Golden brown

Hair:
- ☐ Flaxen blonde
- ☐ Yellow blonde
- ☐ Honey blonde
- ☐ Strawberry blonde (usually with freckles)
- ☐ Strawberry redhead (usually with freckles)
- ☐ Auburn
- ☐ Golden brown
- ☐ Red-black (rare)
- ☐ Dove gray
- ☐ Creamy white

Eyes:
- ☐ Blue with white "rays"
- ☐ Clear blue
- ☐ Steel blue
- ☐ Green with golden flecks
- ☐ Clear green
- ☐ Aqua
- ☐ Teal
- ☐ Golden brown

By now you should know your season. If you want to verify your choice, or if you are still deciding between two seasons, take Step 3 and see yourself in colors. Otherwise, move on and begin putting your colors to use.

The only trick now is emotionally accepting your whole palette—both the colors that are new for you and the missing colors that you have previously worn. The missing colors are gone for two reasons—they upset your wardrobe plan, including your makeup and accessories, and they don't look as good on you as the colors in your palette. Once your eye is adjusted to you in your palette, you will be the first to see that the "old" color doesn't look that good after all. Be open-minded, too, about the new colors in your palette. In class, both the students and I are a support system to convince a hesitant Summer that she really does look great in her fuchsia, or a red-headed Autumn that she can wear red, now that it's the right red.

Now have fun learning more about your color personality. But don't go on a major shopping spree until you've read the rest of the book. You want to be a totally harmonious woman, with your wardrobe, accessories, hair, and makeup just right, before you go out and set the world on fire!

STEP 3: (OPTIONAL): SEEING YOURSELF IN TEST COLORS

First you will try yourself in makeup colors and then you'll drape your neck and shoulders in fabric colors to see which bring out the best in you.

Trying on lipstick and blush colors from opposite seasons is the quickest way to reveal whether your skin tone is warm or cool. (You may use lip gloss and any type of blusher on your cheeks. Even if you prefer not to wear makeup, this test is invaluable in helping you accurately determine your season. Because *many* of the women who come to my classes are wearing the wrong color lipstick, and because your eye is accustomed to seeing whatever makeup you have been wearing to date, you may want to ask a friend or a salesperson to help.

When you try on these colors, wear an off-white shirt or something in a pale neutral so your eye will not judge the color in relation to your clothing. Do not wear any foundation on your face, as you want your skin to show its natural tone.

Now try on the lip and cheek colors that apply to the seasons in question for you. Most department or drug stores have plenty of testers available, or perhaps you have some of these colors floating around your household. Use the following chart as a guide:

		Lipstick	*Blush*
For the Cool Seasons	WINTER	Medium to Dark Pink/Plum or True Red (no orange tones)	Burgundy or Plum
	SUMMER	Light to Medium Pink/Rose	Rose or Pink
For the Warm Seasons	AUTUMN	Terra-Cotta Orange-Red	Dark Peach or Russet
	SPRING	Light Peach, Coral, or Coral-Pink	Peach or Salmon

When you study what each lipstick/blush combination does to your skin, always *compare*. One color may look good, but its opposite may look *better*.

The Winter usually needs color and will look decidedly better in pink or plum than in orange tones. Olive-skinned Winters may be accustomed to wearing peach, but try a deep pink and see the difference! Autumn is the only one who will look good in orange. Summer will usually find the Winter tester too strong, though not always. But she will definitely look better in either of the pink testers than in the orange. She will not look terrible in Spring's peach, but she will look better in pink. Spring wears a peach or coral best of all. Autumn's orange will be too harsh and muted for Spring, even though it is a warm color.

Now it's time to see yourself draped in colors. A solid color scarf, blouse, sheet, towel, or even paper will do. Avoid prints. Use the colors of the printed palettes as guides.

This test is based on comparison. You should compare one color against another, perhaps several times, to see which is better. You may need to compare several sets of colors until you get a clear feeling for the season that is most in harmony with you.

First, there are a few rules you should follow to make the test accurate.

1. Find a place with plenty of natural daylight. You can't see the subtleties of color in dim lighting or under fluorescent light. (I am often asked by well-meaning people to analyze their season at a party over candlelight. Alas, only a magician can do this trick!)

2. Cover your clothes with a large white shirt or sheet. It is extremely distracting for the untrained eye to judge one color while another color is competing for attention.

3. If you dye or color your hair in any way, cover it with an off-white scarf. The eye will look at color plus hair, rather than color plus skin. You want to see what the test colors do to your skin only.

Most people who have trouble determining a season are those whose hair is colored or frosted. (There's no harm in trying on wigs, if you can find any. I keep four on hand in my classroom: neutral brown for Winters and brunette Summers, auburn for Autumns and Springs, ash blonde for blonde Summers, and golden blonde for Springs.)

4. Ask at least two other people (preferably three or four) to do this test with you. One person is not enough because her (or his) opinion may be influenced by personal color preferences rather than by how the color looks on you. Undoubtedly you have co-workers, neighbors, club members, or family who can spare a few minutes to share opinions. (If you must do this test by yourself in front of a mirror, then switch the colors back and forth, allowing each to settle for a minute until you have a clear feeling which group is best.)

5. Gather whichever colors you need to make your comparisons. Use the printed colors on pages 29-35 as guidelines.

6. Try to divorce yourselves from your personal favorite and least favorite colors while observing each other. You are not judging the color, but rather its effectiveness in revealing skin tone. When holding the test colors under your face, you must remember one all-important rule:

LOOK AT THE FACE, NOT AT THE COLOR.

Remember, this is a test based on comparison. One color may look good, but its opposite may look better. Always ask, "Which is better?"

Here's what you look for as you hold a color to your face:

The Right Color:	The Wrong Color:
Smooths and clarifies your complexion; minimizes lines, shadows, and circles; brings a healthy color to your face. Your face will pop out, pushing the color into the background.	May make your complexion look pale, sallow, or "muddy"; will accentuate lines or shadows around the mouth and nose, dark circles under the eyes; will accentuate blotches, if any; may age your face; will look too strong or too weak. The color tends to pop out, pushing your face into the background.

Now compare the colors of the two seasons you have picked from Steps 1 and 2. If you are deciding between a warm and a cool season you must do the test without lipstick or your eye will be influenced by the color on your lips.

AUTUMN or WINTER
Rust or Blue-Red
Warm Beige or Pure White
Dark Brown or Navy Blue
Orange or Magenta

SUMMER or SPRING
Burgundy or Light Orange
Rose-Brown or Golden Brown
Blue-Green or Yellow-Green
Rose-Pink (Blue) or Peach

AUTUMN or SPRING
Mustard or Light Clear Gold
Dark Brown or Golden Brown
Bright Orange or Light Peach
Moss Green or Pastel Yellow-Green

SUMMER or WINTER
Rose-Brown or Black (with makeup)
Soft White or Pure White
Powder Pink or Magenta
Medium Blue or Royal Blue

AUTUMN or SUMMER	WINTER or SPRING
Rust or Blue-Red	Burgundy or Orange-Red
Camel or Rose-Brown	Pure White or Ivory
Orange or Powder Pink	Black or Camel
Moss Green or Blue-Green	Magenta or Peach

Now, try out your season by wearing something you already own in one of your season's colors, being careful to use the appropriate makeup shades. Take yourself someplace where your friends and acquaintances can see you. Their compliments will confirm your choice!

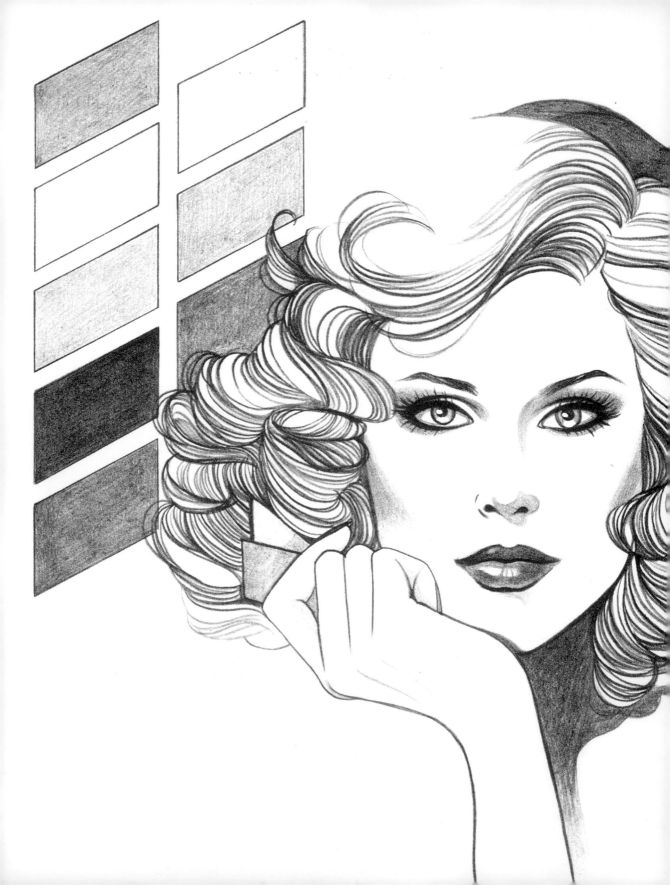

5

YOUR COLOR PERSONALITY: Understanding Your Palette

I ONCE MET A DELICATE SPRING, OF GRANDMOTHERLY AGE YET retaining a youthful quality as Springs often do. She appeared at her first session of my class in powder blue, looking soft, feminine, and dainty, entirely in tune with her personality even though powder blue was not her perfect color. After receiving her spring colors, she returned to class the following week in a wild Indian print dress sporting every bright color in the spring palette! She had clearly misinterpreted her colors.

Your colors work best when you use them to harmonize with your coloring, your body type, and your personality. Our Spring, for example, with her flaxen hair, pale blue eyes, and ivory complexion, had a soft appearance. To achieve her best look, she needed to build her wardrobe around her delicate to medium colors, using only the merest touches of bright as accents. The geometric Indian print was out of character for her.

Within your palette you must choose the colors and combinations that suit you as an individual. Each of the palettes contains both soft and vivid colors, all of which are valuable to you in planning your wardrobe. But some of you may feel most comfortable with a soft image; others may love their bright colors best; and still others prefer to dress in neutrals. Further, your moods may change from year to year. So use your palette ro reflect your own personality, knowing that all your colors are flattering.

Bear in mind, too, that the coloring of people within each season varies in intensity. Most people wear all their colors well, but some, depending on their hair color or the depth of their skin tone, wear some colors best near the face, saving others for accessories or clothing farther from the face. If you are quite fair, for example, you may find that a few of the brightest or darkest colors in your palette are too strong to wear in a large splash near your face. You can still wear these colors, but you should use them in prints, accents, skirts, pants, or accessories. A blazer in one of your dark or bright colors would look best if softened by a blouse in a lighter shade. In contrast, the woman with stronger coloring may find her palest colors or neutrals a little weak, and she should keep her brightest shades near her face and the softer ones in the blazer, skirt, or accessories. With a suntan, a fair person can usually wear her vivid colors.

Now it's time to try on your colors and decide how to use them to your best advantage. Begin by cutting out the printed swatches for your season and placing them in a plastic wallet organizer to keep safely tucked in your purse. The neutrals are arranged together, and the color families are together. Now go on a looking spree, not to buy, but to hold up colors to yourself. Start with your own closet, your family's clothes, and then the stores. Remember, at this point you are just looking in order to understand you color "personality."

Pay special attention to your neutral and basic colors. These will become the backbone of your wardrobe, as they are the ones you will use for a basic coat, suit, and dress. You will usually find some of your neutrals more exciting than others, depending on your hair and eye color. A gray-haired Winter, for example, is especially attractive in a gray coat, while a brunette may be better in navy, using her gray for pants and skirts. When her hair turns gray, she can switch.

You will not find all your colors at once. The fashion industry promotes some colors every year, but most come in cycles. Also, your season's colors are usually easiest to find during "your" season, as this is when these colors fill the stores. But your colors last a lifetime, so eventually you'll have an opportunity to try them all. As I mentioned earlier, your skin tone doesn't change, but it does fade with age. You will not change your palette, but you will draw from your own softer colors once you've become a great-granny. By the same token, if you are sixteen, you may want to save your sophisticated shades for later. You are lucky to find your colors so young!

The colors you are trying on will always look best when you are wearing the correct makeup. Even if you dislike makeup, I strongly suggest that you wear blush. It can be applied to look natural, and you will look healthier and prettier with a little color on your cheeks.

As you "color shop," try to develop an impression of your color self in your mind. Familiarize yourself thoroughly with your colors so that when you shop later for clothes, you will understand your palette. In the future, a "new" color may appear on the fashion scene, one that is not printed in your palette. When you've lived in your palette a while and gotten to know your color self, you will know when a new fashion color is for you. For example, if one year the featured burgundy is a shade with lots of brown in it, bringing it close to mahogany, then an Autumn may wear it. It must be brown enough to go with Autumn's lipstick and accessories.

The charts on pages 66-69 and the descriptions that follow are to be used along with your printed swatches to give you an additional way to conceptualize your season. These are your guidelines when you shop "for real" later.

The swatches themselves are to be used as a guide, not as an absolute. Color printed on paper is less true than color in fabric. You do not have to match the swatches exactly, except where specifically mentioned in the following descriptions. For most colors, you may use your range of, say, greens, held against the garment in question to see if it blends. If it doesn't, it's not for you.

WINTER

You are best in clear colors and sharp contrasts. A Winter strives to stay snappy and should *never* wear muted, powdered tones. When shopping, think *true, blue,* and *vivid; sharp, clear,* and *icy.*

Winter is the only season who successfully wears pure white or black. Don't be afraid of a white blouse; white is exciting on you. Winter's grays range from icy to charcoal; and true gray is yours, but not blue-gray or yellow-gray. (A few gray-haired Winters can wear blue-gray.) Your beige *must* be taupe (gray-beige), always light and clear. You are not a beige person in general and should avoid all rose-beiges and yellow-beiges. Darker taupe may be used for accessories such as shoes and bags. Navy blue is excellent on you, as is burgundy. You may wear any shade of navy, but keep your burgundy bright. You will not look your best in muted maroon tones.

Winter excels in true and primary colors, as well as their bluer and darker counterparts. You wear true red and any blue-red, but not orange-red. Your greens range from true green to emerald to pine, which has a blue cast rather than the yellow cast of Autumn's forest green. True blue, royal blue, hot turquoise, and Chinese blue as well as navy make up your blue family. Royal purple is great, as are hot pinks, from shocking pink to magenta to fuchsia. You have only one shade of yellow: clear, bright lemon. Avoid golden yellow.

Icy tones make the Winter woman sparkle. These are your version of pastels, almost white with a drop of color. You wear icy blue, icy aqua, icy pink, icy violet, icy green, and icy yellow as well as icy versions of your other colors, such as gray and taupe. Avoid all powdered pastels, as they will dull you.

The very fair-skinned Winter is best in the icy and deep colors. The shocking colors are too vivid in large amounts, and she should wear them as accents or away from the face. Deep hot pink, for example, will be better on her than shocking pink. True, emerald, or pine green is better than light true green; blue-red and burgundy are better than true red, and so forth. Fair Winters may also find soft white better than pure white and should soften black near the face. They should mix black with other colors, or wear a scoop neck, letting their skin do the softening. By contrast, some Winters are especially good in the true, bright colors and weak in the palest neutrals, such as gray and beige. Such Winters should use these neutrals in prints or mix them with a brighter color near the face.

If you are a Winter you should never wear orange, gold, rust, peach, orange-reds, yellow-greens, or most beiges and browns. You may wear brown if it is so dark that it can be worn with black accessories. Avoid all muted, dull tones. Stick closely to your color swatches when shopping for your yellow and your taupe. You may deviate from the other swatches up or down a shade.

SUMMER

Summer is the pastel woman and the woman who wears soft neutrals especially well. You should think *blue, rose,* and *soft.* Even though you may be a Summer who favors her bright colors, you should think of yourself as feminine,

Text continues on page 70

COMPARE THE COLORS OF THE FOUR SEASONAL PALETTES.

	WINTER	*SUMMER*
White	Pure White	Soft White
Beige	Gray-Beige (Taupe) Icy Taupe	Rose-Beiges

Gray	True Grays, from Icy
	    to Charcoal
		Blue-Grays
		    Light to Medium

Brown	No Brown No Tan	Rose-Browns Cocoa
Black	Black	No Black
Navy	Any Navy	Grayed Navy
Blue	True Blue Royal Blue Icy Blue	Gray-Blue (including Denim) Sky Blue Periwinkle Blue Powder to Medium Blue
Turquoise	Hot Turquoise Chinese Blue Icy Aqua	Pastel Aqua
Green	Light True Green True Green Emerald Green Icy Green	Blue-Greens, Pastel to Deep

AUTUMN	SPRING
Oyster White	Ivory
Earth Beiges Gold-tone Beiges, including Camel	Clear Beiges Creamy Beiges, including Camel
No Gray	Warm (Yellow) Grays, Light to Medium

Dark Brown,
    Most Browns and Tans
    Coffee, Bronze, Mahogany
	Golden Browns,
	    Clear Tans

No Black	No Black
No Navy	Light Clear Navy
Teal Blue Deep Periwinkle	Light Royal Blue Periwinkle Blues, Light to Dark
Turquoise	Medium Warm Turquoise Clear Aquas

Grayed Yellow-Greens
Yellow-Greens,
    Lime to Bright
Earth Greens,
    Olive, Moss, Jade, Forest
	Clear Yellow-Greens,
	    Pastel to Bright
	
	(Cont'd.)

	WINTER	SUMMER
Orange	No Orange	No Orange
Pink	Shocking Pink Deep Hot Pink (Blue) Magenta, Fuchsia Icy Pink	All Pastel Pinks (Blue) Deep Rose Blue-Pinks
Red	True Red Blue-Reds	Watermelon Blue-Reds Raspberry

Burgundy	Bright Burgundy	Burgundy,
		    including Maroons
		    and Cordovans

Gold	No Gold	No Gold
Yellow	Clear Lemon Yellow Icy Yellow	Light Lemon Yellow
Purple	Royal Purple Icy Violet	Plum Soft Fuchsia Mauve, Orchid, Lavender

AUTUMN	SPRING
All Oranges	Light Oranges
Deep Peach, Salmon	Apricot, Peach, Salmon
Rust, Terra Cotta	All Corals, Light Rust
No Pink	All Peachy (Yellow) Pinks
Orange-Reds	Clear Red
Bittersweet	Orange-Reds
Dark Tomato	
No Burgundy	No Burgundy
All Golds	Clear Gold
Yellow-Gold	Bright Golden Yellow
No Purple	Medium Violet
	Blue-Violet

Continued from page **65**

looking more for softness than for sharp contrast. On you the pastels look strong and vibrant enough.

Soft white (with no yellow) is Summer's best white. Ironically, this is the shade called "winter white" in the stores. Your beige and brown always have a rose tone. Wear any shade between your rose-beige and rose-brown swatches, including cocoa, but avoid yellow-beiges, gray-beiges, and dark browns. You can wear grays from very light blue-gray to any soft charcoal blue-gray.

You are in your territory in most blues, eliminating only the royal or Chinese shades of Winter. Your swatches for blues are simply guides. Keep your aqua light to medium, and your navy grayer and softer than the strong navy of Winter. Grayed navy brings out the beauty of your softer complexion. Blue-greens, ranging from pastel to deep, also belong to Summer, as do all pastel pinks with a blue undertone. You may carry your pinks into deep rose tones, including fuchsia, but often they are best when powdered or muted. Your reds, like your grays and greens, have blue tones. Your watermelon leans a bit toward coral, but you should avoid orange or orange-reds.

The whole family of lavender, orchid, and mauve pastels belongs to Summer. All of them are for you. In addition, you have the darker tones of plum, burgundy, and raspberry, though fair Summers may need to keep a softer shade near the face.

Summer has only one flattering shade of yellow: light lemon. You should stick closely to your yellow swatch and avoid gold tones.

The very fair blonde Summer should soften her darkest colors, such as plum, dark burgundy, and maroon with a lighter color close to her face. The dark brunette Summer is especially good in the vivid colors of her palette and may find that the palest pastels are best mixed with brighter colors. She is the woman who just missed being a Winter.

All Summers should avoid black, pure white, yellow-beige, gold, orange, yellow-greens, and all yellow undertones. Black may be used as an accessory in shoes and bags. With a tan, a Summer woman may get away with pure white, but it is still too strong a look for your overall soft image. You do not want to look sharp around the edges.

AUTUMN

You Autumns have the easiest shopping! Your colors are readily available. And because you can wear either muted or clear tones, you needn't be too careful in matching your swatches. You may use your swatches as a general guide, except for your blues, where you should stick to your printed samples. Always think of golden undertones when you shop.

Your best white is oyster, a beige-tone white. You wear all warm beiges, from light to dark, except taupe (gray-beige) and rose-beige. Dark chocolate brown is especially exciting on you, though you wear all browns well—mahogany, camel, tan, and bronze tones. Any gold, yellow-gold, pumpkin, mustard, or terra cotta is good. Your oranges range from medium peach and muted salmon to bright orange and rust. Orange-reds and bittersweet reds are your best. Yellow-greens, from grayed to bright, and earth greens, from jade to moss, are for you. Forest green is especially becoming. Be careful with your blues. Your turquoise and teal are strong and muted, and your periwinkle is deep.

The very fair Autumn may be overwhelmed by the strength of the brightest colors, such as orange, chartreuse, bright yellow-green, and turquoise. She is best in the soft or muted colors, the neutrals, peach, periwinkle, and jade. By contrast, a dark-skinned Autumn may look a little drab in the muted earth colors of this palette. She needs to wear her bright colors closest to her face, saving the muted ones for skirts and shoes, or to mix in prints. She needs makeup to look her best in beige and softer colors.

All Autumns should avoid black, pink, navy, gray, blue-reds, and all colors with blue undertones. Be careful that your peach, periwinkle, and lime green are not too pale.

SPRING

Springs are the most delicate of all the seasons, yet they need colors that are alive. When you shop, think *clear, warm* (yellow), and *crisp.* Your colors are the hardest to find, because they must be clear, never muted, and not too dark. Because of your delicate beauty, you remain ageless—a compensation for having to search a little harder for your colors.

Spring's best white is ivory, a creamy tone, though you may also wear off-white. Your beiges are all clear and warm—from light beige to camel. Your browns begin with golden tan and go as dark as milk chocolate; any golden brown is good as long as it is not too dark. Spring has clear golds, from buff to golden yellow, bright but not harsh.

Only one shade of gray is flattering to Spring: warm (yellow) gray, in a light shade if near the face. Spring's navy blue is light navy, clear and bright. Dark navy is harsh and aging. Stick closely to your gray and navy swatches when shopping.

Spring has many shades of aqua and clear turquoise, and these are especially good on you. You are also vibrant in light true blue, periwinkle blue, from light to dark, and medium violet. Although Spring is often accustomed to wearing powder blue, you are not as exciting in it as you are in your periwinkle shades. Periwinkle has more violet in it, which brings Spring to life.

Peach, apricot, salmon, and coral, as well as all peachy pinks, are for Spring. You may wear any light orange, bright coral, and orange-red. You are good in clear red, but must avoid blue-reds. Yellow-greens are for you as long as they are clear. Your greens range from pastel to bright.

The very fair, delicate Spring is overpowered by too much of her brightest colors, such as bright golden yellow, bright yellow-green, and sometimes clear red and violet. For her, these are accent colors, good as a sash around a sun hat or in beach clothes or funwear. By contrast, the Spring with stronger coloring looks great in a whole dress of bright yellow-green or golden yellow, but she looks pale in her lightest colors and sometimes in camel. These are best when mixed or used as accessories. This Spring may also add a clear, light rust, and a bright, clear teal or peacock blue to her palette.

If you are a Spring you should avoid black, pure white, colors with blue undertones, dark and muted colors. You may wear black in prints, unless you are very fair.

COMMONLY ASKED QUESTIONS

There are three questions I am inevitably asked in my classes:

1. *Could I be more than one season?*

The answer is no. You will look *best* in one palette; your wardrobe coordinates in one palette; and your makeup goes with one palette. Further, each palette has its own personality. As you grow into your season you develop a special image. You will defeat the purpose of your colors if you adopt two seasons.

Occasionally a woman of redheaded complexion can combine the Autumn and Spring colors, removing colors that are too strong or those that clash with her hair. Her makeup and accessories will blend because the seasons are both warm. She should call herself an Autumn, even though she will be wearing some Spring colors.

2. *Why can't I wear black if I'm not a Winter?*

Black is too strong for all but a Winter. Blonde hair will look blonder, but your face will be overpowered and less beautiful in black. People will see your blonde hair and black dress before they notice *you*. If black turns you on, why not wear it in the bedroom? It's a wonderfully sexy color.

3. *What if I'm in the wrong season?*

You'll know very quickly. Mistakes usually occur only on the person who colors or frosts her hair.

Wear the colors of the season you think you are for one week, drawing from clothes you already own and using the appropriate makeup. Listen for compliments and ask your friends. If it isn't working, do the same with your second season. If you color your hair, go to a wig shop and try on hair colors.

Repeat the original test if necessary, including Step 3.

Now that you know your color personality and understand your palette, let's move on to your clothing personality. Your colors and your type are the most important aspects of selecting clothing to express and complement the real you.

6

YOUR CLOTHING PERSONALITY: *What Type Are You?*

WHAT WORD COMES TO MIND WHEN YOU THINK OF THE FOLLOWING movie and stage personalities? Cher, Carol Burnett, Sandy Duncan, Liz Taylor? For me, Cher is dramatic; Carol Burnett, funny and down-to-earth; Sandy Duncan, a pixie; Liz Taylor, sexy. Perhaps you have different reactions, but you will probably agree that each of these women has a type. Picture Cher in a dramatic halter-top gown with a diamond-shaped cutout exposing her navel. Looks terrific—on her. Now imagine Carol Burnett appearing in the same gown. Ridiculous? Of course. And wouldn't Sandy Duncan look out of character in Liz's low-cut satin?

Your clothing personality—the type or "flavor" in clothing that is best for you—is partially determined by your season because your palette has a certain personality of its own.

A Winter, with her dark (or white) hair and deep eyes, tends toward the dramatic. Looking at the Winter palette, you can see that these colors have a dramatic, sophisticated, perhaps formal, quality, calling for clothes with sleek, clean lines. Her prints must have value contrast and are best worn away from the face, with the exception of small scarves. The Winter is usually best in solids, for her palette's striking colors speak for themselves. The Summer palette has classic colors, reflecting calmness and conservatism, and the Summer woman is most often a poised, gracious, even-tempered person, ideal in classic clothes and soft prints. She's the elegant, but feminine type.

Autumn's palette speaks of warmth and friendliness. The Autumn woman is probably the natural, informal person, best in casual, sporty clothes. She's good in paisleys, plaids, and casual, colorful prints. The colors in Spring's palette are lively, bright, and youthful. Spring herself is often a friendly, informal, bubbly person who never seems to age and has a girlish, feminine quality even in her clothes. Her prints are crisp and colorful, but delicate in feeling.

But what if you are a Winter who is tiny, with rounded features and an innocent, youthful quality—not dramatic at all? Or perhaps you're a Spring who is five feet nine inches tall, with an athletic build, captain of the local soccer team. You may have delicate, youthful coloring, but you certainly would not look your best dressed in girlish ruffles.

Determining the personality in clothing that best suits you depends on more than your season. Your type derives, in addition, from your facial features, height, and bone structure.

It's time to study yourself in the mirror again, this time in a full-length mirror. If you don't have one, put it on your priority list. A full-length mirror is your most honest friend and the only way to get a realistic view of yourself.

Stand in front of the mirror and look first at your face. Do you have even, regular features or a prominent nose or chin or perhaps high cheekbones? Do you have a square jaw? Big eyes? A turned-up nose?

Now check out your body. Is your neck long, short, or average? Are your shoulders square, sloped, or average? Are they broad or narrow? Are you buxom or flat or somewhere in the middle? Is your waist anything special in either direction? How about your hips? Round? Flat? Are your legs long, short, average?

Let's see how your body and features help you arrive at the best look for you. The sooner you understand and accept your body type, the happier you will be. Trying to wear high-style, boy-cut clothes when your figure is shaped like an hourglass only results in disappointment. You will look your best when you dress to enhance what you are instead of trying to be what you are not. Make the most of your uniqueness!

FASHION TYPES
To illustrate the differences among types, we'll identify dramatic, natural, gamin, romantic, ingenue, and classic. In addition, we'll take a look at business attire for all types. These images are not absolutes and they may overlap, but you will see how each type influences the selection of clothes, makeup, hair style, and accessories.

Dramatic
The woman who wears the dramatic look well is usually tall and thin, with dark or striking coloring and angular features. Any sharp or prominent facial feature is great on a dramatic. So are broad, even bony, shoulders. (See how you can turn your least favorite qualities into assets?) If you aren't tall, but have

dramatic features, you may dress dramatically in touches, but not all over. Full-fledged dramatics are skinny and exotic-looking and have flat hips and long legs.

The dramatic type wears extremes in fashion—either straight lines and hard-finish fabrics or ultra billowy clothes. If you are dramatic, you may wear severely plain or lavishly ornate fabrics and styles. Wear the most exotic colors in your palette, including neutrals in shiny solids or glittery weaves. Your prints are bold, wild, vivid, or ethnic in geometrics, paisleys, or stylized designs. For dressy occasions, you can wear satin, crepe, heavy brocade, or metallics—any theatrical or striking fabric or texture.

Because of your height, you can add emphasis at the waist or even below, such as dangling belts or lavish trim on a hemline. Your jewelry should be bold, simple, and large, or elaborate and ornate. Your hair, too, may be severely simple (short or long), ornately curled, or sleeked back in a chignon. Makeup applied theatrically works for you, for dramatics are not conservative types. On you almost anything goes.

Dramatics are usually Winters or dark Autumns. Most Summers and Springs who are tall and angular are best to go for a sophisticated rather than a dramatic look. It's just too severe for their softer coloring. Typical dramatics are Cher, Diana Ross, Lauren Bacall, and Barbra Streisand.

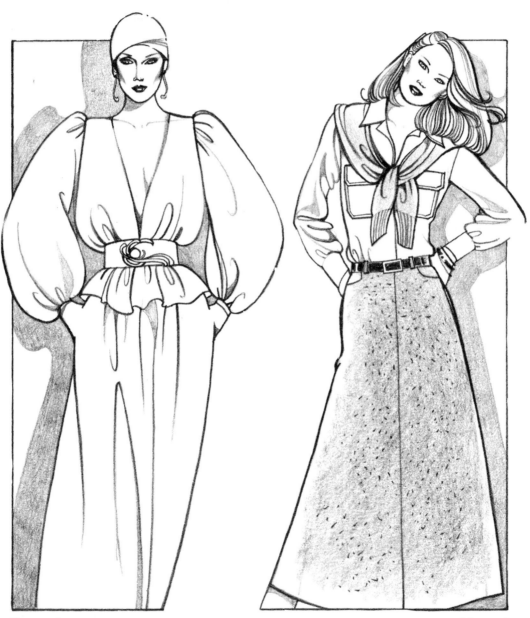

Dramatic   *Natural*

Natural

The natural woman is the casual type. Often she has wide-set eyes and a squarish jaw. She is usually tall and may be athletic, but even if she's not, she has an energetic stride and an informal, friendly manner.

If you are a natural, you look good in all kinds of sportswear, from casual to chic. You can wear boots and leather, skirts and sweaters, tailored suits with top-stitching, or unconstructed jackets. A mix-and-match wardrobe works well for you since separate clothing pieces and pattern combinations suit you. Nubby, natural, and hand-woven fabrics are good, as are tweeds, plaids, checks, and paisleys. Your prints should be large, casual designs. Solids are great for you too, especially in textured fabrics, such as heavy crepe, raw silk, jersey, even quilted material. All natural types should avoid shiny fabrics.

The natural woman is best in simple jewelry and not much of it. Makeup is minimal and natural and hair needs a casual cut and can look windblown.

The Autumn palette lends itself especially well to the natural look, though women of any season can fit this cate-

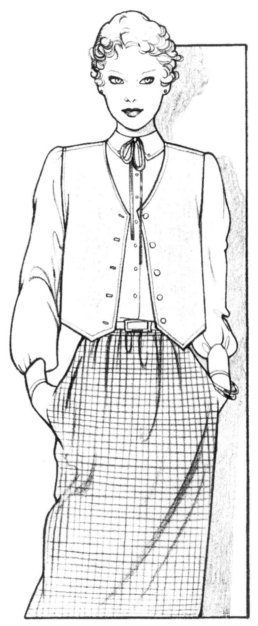

Gamin   © Color Me Beautiful, Inc. 1984

gory. Farrah Fawcett, Ethel Kennedy, Candice Bergen, Carol Burnette, and Katharine Hepburn are the natural type.

Gamin

The petite stature and pixie face of the gamin keep her eternally youthful. Although she is slight in build, the gamin is compact and well-proportioned rather than delicate or dainty. She has a friendly, bubbly personality and a "go-for-it" attitude.

Clean, straight lines and natty details in her clothes complement both her body type and her energetic spirit. Contrasting buttons, patch pockets, a tie or a vest all suit her when scaled down to her size. She can wear ruffles if they are cotton rather than silk and stand-up rather than drape.

Crisp, light-weight fabrics with a matte finish create the snappy, well-pressed appearance that suits her. She can wear tweeds but only if sharp rather than blended. Her prints must be small and defined. Evenly-spaced stripes, checks and small geometrics work well for her.

The gamin's uncluttered look calls for little jewelry, usually no more than small stud earrings, and a moderate amount of makeup. A tight, curly perm works well for some, but a short, straight, sassy cut is also good.

Gamins can be any season, but are most likely to be Winters or Springs. Mary Martin, Goldie Hawn, Sandy Duncan, Judy Carne, and June Allyson all fit the gamin type.

Romantic

Romantic women should seek femininity in both style and fabric. The romantic woman has a curvy figure and looks best in clothes that have gently curved lines, with either a crisply bouffant or a softly draped silhouette. Her fabrics should be luxurious and soft, with a sheen, and her prints should be rounded in feeling and design. Because she has striking coloring, the romantic woman may dress with theatrical flair, though she must take care not to look overdone or gaudy. She may wear exaggerated styles and sophisticated prints as long as they are feminine.

The romantic often has a beautiful face or a special facial feature, such as her eyes or complexion, and should choose necklines, accessories, and accent colors from her palette to draw the eye to her face. She looks beautiful in evening wear, and her rounded figure is shown to its best advantage in a low-cut neckline and, if she's slim, a fitted waist. For evening, she is good in chiffon, silk, lace, shiny satin, brocade, velvet, and many other sophisticated fabrics, simple or ornate.

Jewelry for the romantic woman must be delicate in detail, though it may have a luxurious look. Her hair is best in curves or curls, even if she sweeps it off her face, and her makeup can be strong if it is not overdone. The romantic is often the woman who will take the time to put on false eyelashes.

Romantics come from all the seasons. Elizabeth Taylor and Jaclyn Smith are Winter romantics; Ann-Margret, Autumn; Zsa Zsa Gabor and Marilyn Monroe, Springs; and Peggy Lee, Summer. The romantic look requires maturity, so if you are still in your twenties, dress for femininity, but save the theatrical for later.

Ingenue
The ingenue is the youthful romantic: pretty, dainty, delicate in build and coloring. The ingenue also needs feminine styles, curved lines, soft or crispy fabrics, and delicate prints. She looks good in floral prints, especially those that are animated or outlined. However, she is not theatrical or flamboyant, and her figure is youthful. She looks best in hair styles with curves or curls—soft, loose, or tight. She has a fresh, unsophisticated, natural femininity and should wear dainty jewelry and minimal makeup. She is best in her softer colors and light-weight fabrics with a matte finish. Sheer, crisp cotton, voile, organdy, dotted swiss, eyelet, thin jersey, or any youthful fabric is suitable for evening wear. Heavy, shiny, or glittery fabric is too overpowering for the ingenue.

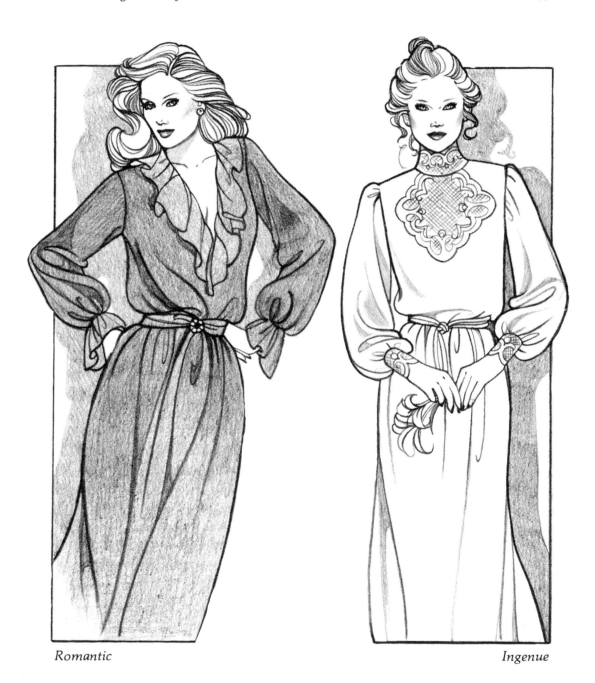

Romantic   Ingenue

The ingenue eventually matures out of this girlish look, usually becoming the more sophisticated romantic or a classic. She never becomes dramatic or sporty. Spring women are most likely to be the ingenue type, and, though a young feminine woman of any season may be an ingenue, Spring seems to stay that way the longest, probably because of her delicate coloring. Helen Hayes, Debbie Reynolds, and Sandra Dee are all Springs who remained ingenues well into their "prime." Sally Struthers is an ingenue maturing into a romantic, while Shirley Jones is more classic. The main point to remember, if you are this type, is that eventually you must give up ruffles and bows for a more mature look.

Classic

If you have even, regular facial features, medium coloring, and a well-proportioned body, you are the classic type. The classic woman is tailored, conservative but smart, always well groomed. Typically, she has good posture, a sense of formality, and poise.

The classic woman avoids extremes in fashion, fabric, and prints. She is a scaled-down dramatic, avoiding trendy

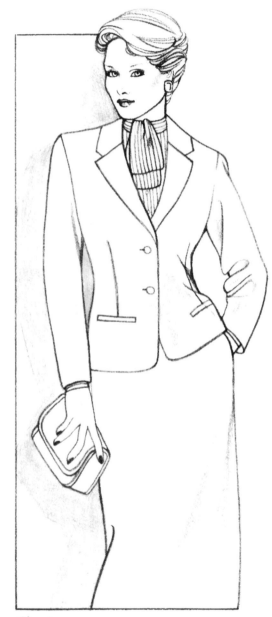

Classic   © Color Me Beautiful, Inc. 1984

fashion and severe, straight lines, but achieving distinction through fine fabric, soft, straight lines, and immaculately tailored clothes. A bouffant or crisp silhouette is not for her. The classic stays up-to-date in a conservative way: her hemlines go up and down just a little and she switches to the latest look only after it has become established.

Fabric for the classic woman may be shiny or matte, but not too heavy. Fine cottons and jerseys, tissue wool and wool crepe, fine knits, and Qiana are all good. Prints, again, must be middle-of-the-road: small to medium, stylized designs, paisley and polka dots or any small pattern that repeats evenly. For a Summer classic, a watercolor effect is also nice. A Spring classic can have a more animated print, perhaps outlined to make it stand out from the fabric. Winter and Autumn classics look good in paisleys, stripes, and conservative geometrics. For dress, the classic is good in chiffon, crepe, silk, tissue fabric, or subtle brocade. A smooth or fine fabric is always better than one with a rough texture.

If you are the classic type, you must choose a controlled hair style that you can keep neat. The casual, windblown look is incompatible with your image. Your hair may be straight or curled, but not extreme. No afro for you unless you are black, because an afro is classic for a black woman. Your makeup, too, must be conservative, but *do* wear makeup. The same is true for your jewelry. It should be of average size, subtle, but smart and chic. And *do* wear jewelry, especially earrings. Because the classic woman is "medium" everything, she must be careful not to look plain, dowdy, or matronly. If you wear enough makeup, jewelry, and accessories to look smart, you can find the classic look exciting.

Although everyone can wear classic clothes, this look does not suit everyone equally. A woman with a dramatic face or body will look boring in classic clothes, while a voluptuous, romantic woman will look severe.

Princess Grace, Dina Merrill, Diahann Carroll, Pat Nixon, and Rosalynn Carter are typical classic women.

Achieving Several Looks

Some women can achieve several looks successfully. Sophia Loren can dress romantically or dramatically with equal credibility. Faye Dunaway can be natural or dramatic. Put her in a softly tailored suit and a short, controlled hair style, and she's classic.

Whatever look you favor, just be sure it is believable on you. When Jackie Kennedy Onassis was the President's wife, her image-makers tried to force her into a classic mold, in tailored suits, pillbox hats, and gloves. She looked constrained. The real Jackie, a natural, emerged in later pictures, perched on the rail of a yacht with her hair blowing in the wind. Pat Nixon, on the other hand, is a true classic, looking her best in softly tailored lines, hair in place.

Of course, some occasions call for you to achieve a certain look—romantic, sporty, or conservative—in order to be dressed appropriately. Then you must adapt the required look to your style. You may be best in classic clothes, but when you're going to a football game you want to look sporty. While a plaid pantsuit would not be right for you, a checkered jacket with solid-color blouse and pants would do the trick. By the same token, your best friend, the cheer-leader type, can wear plaid from head to toe and look terrific.

PRINTS

Your choice of prints and plaids is very important in achieving your look. When selecting them, always scale the design to your size and height. A tall woman would normally wear a large print unless she has a very delicate bone structure, in which case she would be better in a medium-size print. A short woman with a sturdy build would also choose a medium-size print to blend her height with her body structure.

Often a print contains colors from more than one season. You can still buy it as long as you use the following guidelines:

1. The wrong color should not dominate the print.

2. The wrong color should not be too close to your face.

3. The print should not require you to wear accessories, such as shoes, from another palette.

Some women are not their happiest or best in any prints. There's nothing wrong with that. Stick to solids and use jewelry, belts, scarves, or interesting fabrics to add variety to your outfit.

DRESSING FOR BUSINESS

At the office, regardless of your type, classic is best. A business suit or a conservative dress is appropriate, especially while you are striving to establish yourself on the job. Be sure your suit is in one of your colors, however. The popular gray suit theory is fine for Winters and Summers, but an Autumn or Spring in a charcoal gray suit will not create her best impression. You can achieve the same look in your own colors. Keep your makeup and jewelry modest. Be well groomed, but not flamboyant.

Even in a business environment, you can express your individuality as long as you do it conservatively. A dramatic woman can modify her suited look with a longer skirt, heavier jewelry, or a stronger print or color in her blouse. A romantic woman can wear a softer fabric and a blouse of silk with a soft bow rather than a tailored oxford cloth shirt. The natural can choose tweeds and oxford cloth rather than silk. Once you have proven yourself as a budding executive, you can take more liberties in expressing your clothing personality. But never dress too romantically at work unless you are aspiring for the boss rather than a promotion.

If you work in a field concerned with the arts, fashion, or women, you can wear less conservative clothing. You may in fact go further on the staff of a fashion magazine if you dress with style and flair.

YOUR OWN BEST LOOK

Using the following list, check the looks you feel are for you. As you experiment, see which image gets you the most compliments. Check the Sunday newspaper advertisements and clip out looks that you would like to try. One of my students taped these to her mirror to keep in mind the "new person" she was becoming. She has become a veritable fashion plate.

Check the looks that are best for you:

	Me	Not Me	Try it
Styles:			
Severe, straight lines			
Soft, straight lines			
Soft, curved lines			
Bouffant, crisp lines			
Billowy, blousy			
Clingy			
Detail:			
Contrasting trim: piping, buttons			
Crisp stand-up ruffles			
Soft ruffles, flounces			
Pleats			
Soft pleats (folds)			
Bows			
Silk flower			
Lace			
Fur trim			

	Me	Not Me	Try it
Fabric types:			
These could be cotton, wool, polyester, blends, leather, suede—any natural or man-made fiber, including dressy fabrics.			
Shiny			
Matte			
Smooth			
Rough			
Finely textured (weave or knit)			
Nubby (weave or knit)			
Tweedy			
Prints:			
Large			
Medium			
Small			
Bold			
Moderate			
Subtle, blended			

	Me	Not Me	Try it
Defined, crisp			
Sophisticated			
Casual			
From head to toe (dress, suit)			
From waist up or waist down (blouse, jacket, skirt)			

Jewelry:

	Me	Not Me	Try it
Large			
Medium			
Small			
Delicate, simple			
Dainty, but lavish			
Abstract, modern			
Ornate, baroque			
Classic			
Hand-made			

	Me	*Not Me*	*Try it*
Hair:			
Severe			
Ornate			
Casual, windblown			
Soft curls			
Controlled curves			
Tight curls (perm)			
Straight			
High-fashion			
Conservative			
Makeup:			
Minimal			
Moderate			
Elaborate			

Understanding your best clothing personality takes time, awareness, and trial and error. We are usually the last to see ourselves objectively, so be open-minded. Remember, too, to keep abreast of the changes you undergo over the years. You may be an ingenue at nineteen but a classic at thirty. Keep your image appropriate to your age. It isn't fun to dress too old when you're young, and it isn't flattering to dress too young when you're mature.

Explore the personality of clothing, and enjoy finding the look that is *yours*. With your colors and your most flattering image, you are on your way to being a totally beautiful, totally together woman.

Reference:
For further information on clothing personalities, see *Art and Fashion in Clothing Selection,* by Harriett T. McJimsey (Ames: Iowa State University Press, 1973), pp. 69-104.

7

FASHIONS, FIGURES AND FADS

FASHION IS ONLY AS GOOD AS IT LOOKS ON *YOU*. SOME WOMEN seem to be able to wear the latest lines every year, but most of us cannot. The smart woman adapts the latest look to her own figure and personality rather than trying to alter her personal look to accommodate each trend. If you wear a style that doesn't look good on you—even if it's "in"—you do not look stylish.

Now let's turn to your figure and proportions and work on finding your best lines.

To start with, try not to become preoccupied with your flaws, but consider your assets instead. Don't be the woman who wears a jacket that comes down to her knees to cover a big fanny, or the one who refuses to smile and expose her crooked teeth. In the first case, you will look top-heavy and short-legged; in the second, you will look unhappy.

When you see yourself in the mirror, you probably zero in on blemishes, wrinkles, and bulges. All of them will seem to disappear when you learn to put together and project a total look that emphasizes your natural coloring and your best features. The people you meet will see an attractive woman with a warm, genuine smile—not crooked teeth. Besides, perfect is boring.

The object of this chapter is to teach you to achieve that total look. You have learned how to make color work for you. Now you will learn to select the lines and details that best complement *your* figure, proportions, and type.

Let's discuss the ways to deal with various figure problems.

POSTURE:
Your posture dictates how good your clothes look on you; even the most expensive and beautifully fitted garment cannot overcome the unflattering effect of a slouching body. The lines of your clothes will hang gracefully if your shoulders are held erect and your tummy and derriere are tucked in.

Stand straight with your weight distributed evenly on both feet. Imagine a string running from your chest bone to the ceiling, suspending you like a marionette. Now drop your shoulders. Shake your head slightly from side to side. You should now be standing correctly.

Practice standing this way in front of a mirror, looking at yourself from the front and from the side. Practice walking while pulling up through your midriff, head carried high, shoulders down. When you walk, swing your leg from the joint at the hip rather than the knee. This stride is smooth and elegant.

PROPORTION:

Understanding your proportions is the key to dressing yourself to your best advantage. Few of us have the perfect proportions that would allow us to wear almost anything, but we can create the illusion of average proportions by dressing in lines that fool the eye.

Ideally, your shoulders should be just an inch or so wider than your hips to allow the lines of your clothes to fall loosely over the hips from the shoulders. To determine your proportions, stand in stocking feet against a door and ask someone to make tiny pencil marks to indicate where each shoulder bone and hip bone is situated. Measure the distances between the marks. If your hips are more than an inch wider than your shoulders, or vice versa, you can take steps to give the illusion of a better proportion.

Next mark your height; then mark your leg length at the point where your thigh joint "breaks" from the hip. Measure both distances from the floor. The average leg length is half of your entire height. If your measurements reveal a discrepancy of more than an inch either way, you will want to use some camouflage, though slightly long legs are often an advantage. Now, mark the door at your waist and your armpit. The well-positioned waist falls in the middle between your armpit and the leg "break," and a variation of more than an inch defines you as either high-waisted or low-waisted.

Write down these measurements and keep your proportions in mind as we discuss the ways to flatter each part of your body.

Last, look at the size of your head in relation to your body. A small head gives the illusion of height, while a large head shortens. If your head seems too small or too large, adjust your hair style, making it either closer to your face to compensate for a large head or fuller for a small one.

FACIAL SHAPE:

If the shape of your face is extreme in any way, avoid repeating this shape in your neckline. For example, a round face looks rounder in a rounded scoop neck; a square jaw is emphasized by a square neckline; and a long, thin face, especially one with a pointed chin, looks longer in a narrow V-neck. A contrasting neckline balances your face.

NECK:

If your neck is too long, very short hair will accentuate its length. For you, it's best to add some length, at least in back, and avoid deep V necklines. You can wear scarves, mandarin collars, choker necklaces, or ribbons at the throat, and you are the lucky lady who can wear the generally unflattering cowl.

If your neck is short, an open collar, V, or scoop neck is your best. Avoid high or standup collars, turtlenecks, and cowls. A crew or mock turtle-neck will work for you. Short hair is always your best bet, because it creates the illusion of distance between your head and shoulders.

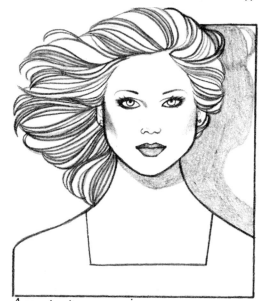

Accentuates square jaw

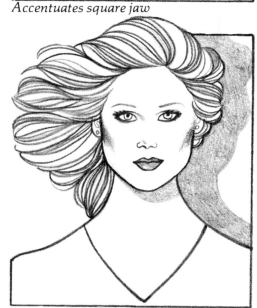

Minimizes square jaw

Even with a short neck, you may wear scarves, but choose a soft fabric and a small size to avoid bulk.

To minimize a wide neck, keep a jewel or crew neckline close to the base of the neck on both sides. A gap on the sides adds width, which is fine for the average or thin neck, but not for you.

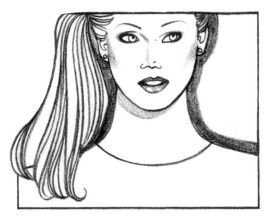
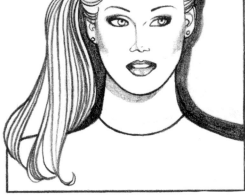

Broadens wide neck   *Minimizes wide neck*

SHOULDERS:
Shoulders come in three general types: square, average-tapered, and sloped.

Any neckline that is horizontal and shallow, such as a bateau, will make your shoulders look broader, and, if they are square, even more square. Conversely, the opposite line—deep and narrow, such as a V—will make shoulders appear narrower and less square. Avoid a halter top if you have either too-broad or too-narrow shoulders, as this line is unflattering to both.

If you have a shoulder problem, you can compensate by using these principles:

Too Broad or Square:

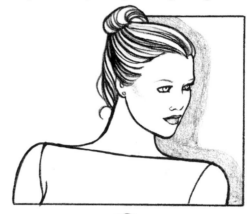

Wide and shallow neckline is unflattering.

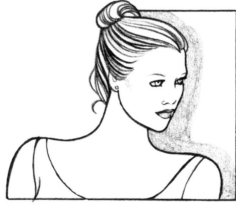

Deep neckline minimizes.

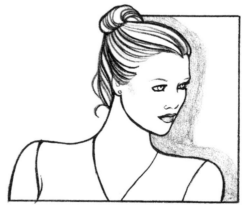

Narrow and deep minimizes.

Too Narrow or Sloped:

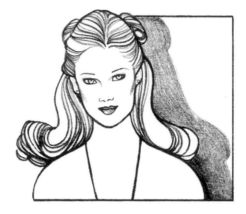

Narrow and deep neckline is unflattering.

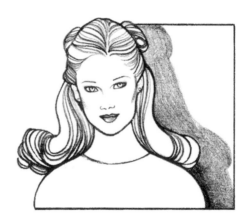

Shallow neckline minimizes.

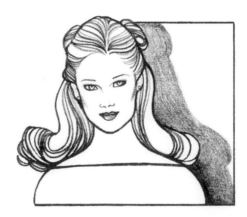

Wide and shallow draws the eyes out.

A lapel is always more flattering than a plain neckline if your shoulders are not your best feature. Lapels that point up and out broaden the shoulder, while lapels that point down narrow them. Buy whichever kind is appropriate for you. Scale the size of your lapels to the size of your body. A large lapel on a tiny body is overwhelming, but a flouncy collar that extends over the shoulder bones is flattering to all shoulders and is appropriate even for the small woman if the fabric is not bulky.

Raglan   *Kimono*

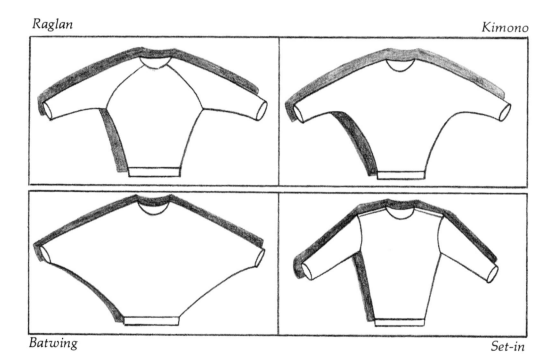

Batwing   *Set-in*

Your shoulder seam is extremely important in creating the illusion of a good shoulder. A *set-in* sleeve is most flattering and can be adjusted to create a slimmer or wider look, depending on your need. For the broad or square shoulder, keep the placement of the shoulder seam right on the shoulder bone.

You may even cheat by moving the seam in a quarter inch if you have enough fullness in the sleeve to allow arm room. The overweight woman can look slimmer in clothes with a crisp, narrow shoulder line and judicious placement of the shoulder seam.

Your shoulder treatment affects the look of your entire silhouette. For the sloped or narrow shoulder, let the seam extend a bit beyond your shoulder bone, to widen. The seam will also give your shoulders the definition of shape they may lack. A woman with a very large bust also may use this trick to call attention away from her bust and draw the eye up and out.

Such sleeve styles as batwing, kimono, and raglan require a broad or squarish shoulder. The raglan, especially, tends to drop the shoulder downward, so women with sloping or narrow shoulders should avoid this line. It is even chancy on shoulders with an average taper, though you can alter the line of these styles by adding a lapel or collar that points up or out.

In sleeveless tops you should follow the same principle as with the shoulder seam. Keep the edge of the garment on the shoulder bone for broad or square shoulders, slightly beyond the bone for narrow or sloped. A sleeveless top with the line inside the bone will accentuate either problem. This line is best for the woman with good, average shoulders.

Any detail on a shoulder will broaden or accentuate it. Epaulets, for example, should be removed from your outfit if you wish to minimize your shoulders, but they are great for adding dimension to shoulders that are too narrow, assuming an epaulet is your type.

There is no such thing as a right or wrong shoulder line, simply whatever is right or wrong for *you*! Remember, you are creating balance. Look in the mirror and ask, "Do my shoulders balance my hips?" Perhaps the upward-pointed lapel is okay because it is balanced by pockets on the hips or by a skirt with some fullness. The exception is the overweight woman, whose hips usually are wider than her shoulders and arms. She does best to create a "slim" shoulder look rather than extending her shoulders to balance her hips. Later, after she loses weight, she can compensate for a too-narrow shoulder, if that becomes her problem.

Don't be afraid to be creative. Your tailor or your sewing machine has the power to improve the line of your outfit. Remove or add shoulder detail, change the direction of a collar, or change the placement of a shoulder seam. These are *not* difficult alterations, but do remember that you may need to lengthen a cuff if you're nipping in a shoulder.

ARMS:
To determine whether your arm is long, average, or short, let your arm hang at your side, and look in the mirror. If your first knuckle aligns with your crotch, you have an average arm. Your elbow should be at your waist.

A wide cuff at the wrist shortens the look of your arm. If your arms are long, this is great; if they're short, avoid wide cuffs. A woman with long arms often has trouble finding sleeves that are long enough. Don't overlook the possibility of adding a cuff, even in a contrasting color.

Everyone can wear a long sleeve, but the three-quarter sleeve looks best on a short woman or one with short arms. It is unflattering on long arms, on a woman with large hands, and on a tall woman who wants to minimize her height.

The short sleeve usually looks best if it falls one inch above or below the bust-line, rather than right at the point of the bust. (If you are small-busted, it may not matter, however.) A sleeve ending just above the elbow can look matronly, especially if it has a rolled cuff or if your arms are heavy. In high-style clothing, this sleeve length can be attractive if you are slim and tall with average to long arms.

If your arms are heavy, avoid long sleeves that are tight or clingy—this accentuates fat.

BUST:
Your bra can make or break the line of your outfit. Braless is fine for the woman with a youthful bust, but for the rest of us a bra is sexier and smoother. When you are wearing a bra, your nipple should be no more than three inches below your armpit (unless you are *very* full-busted). Take a good look at yourself to be sure your bra is doing its job. It may not be.

Many women make the mistake of buying the cup too small and the band too large. Get the snuggest fit around your rib cage that is comfortable, and the largest cup that still fits smoothly. In addition, women are built either far apart or close together, and bras are designed in both fashions. Be sure you are buying a brand cut for you.

If your bust is very small, you will have to avoid necklines intended to show cleavage. But take heart. It is much easier to dress a small bust than a large one. You can wear high-style clothes and all the wonderful blousy designs that the large-busted woman must avoid. Be grateful for small blessings.

There is no escaping the fact that a large bust is a difficult figure problem, partly because it is hard to find clothes that fit. Here are some tips for the busty lady:

- Avoid sleeve lengths ending at the bust.

- Avoid horizontal lines at bust level—no seam, stripe, piping, or similar detail.

- Avoid a low yoke (or smocking) at the bustline.

- Try garments that taper gently under the bustline. Too much fullness adds bulk, and an outfit that is too fitted will accentuate your bust. Pass up a peasant blouse, which makes the figure fuller, in favor of a tailored blouse, which makes it slimmer. It is worthwhile to tailor or alter garments by adding a seam under the bustline, thus slimming the midriff, removing excess fullness, and adding the illusion of length between the waist and bust.

- Avoid high-waisted looks.

- Keep your belts small and, if possible, the same color as your skirt or dress. A self belt is good.

- Wear your collars open, and wear V necklines with lapels, rather than high necklines with no detail, such as turtlenecks or crew necks. Vertical lines— a necklace, a seam, a slit, small buttons—all help to minimize a large bustline.

WAIST:

If you have a small waist, you're the lucky one who can have fun with belts. But if your tiny waist is in the middle of an hourglass figure—with large bust and hips—take care not to look too nipped-in or you will accentuate those other features. A gentle taper, with perhaps a tie belt, is your best look.

If your waist is wide, there's no point in calling attention to it. Use belts judiciously, keeping them narrow and the same color or fabric as the garment. Or simply have a seam at the waist with no belt. Look for princess styles or high- or low-waisted dresses. Make use of the no-waist look with an overblouse or perhaps a second layer such as a loose vest or sweater.

A short-waisted woman is also wise to use a narrow self belt or no belt. If your waist is high, you need to leave as much room as possible between your bust and your waistline. For you, a gentle taper under the bustline is effective in lengthening your midriff. When you wear separates, choose your belt to match your top, rather than your skirt or pants. This trick adds length to your waist. Skirts and pants cut without a waistband are your best bet.

For a long waist, do the opposite. Unless your waist is large, use wide belts that match the color of your skirt, thus bringing the eye up. Choose skirts and pants with waistbands, including high-waisted bands. You can also cheat a little with your waist seams, raising them half an inch or so above your real waistline.

HIPS:

Narrow hips allow you to wear high-style designs and any boy-cut fashion. But if your hips are considerably narrower than your shoulders, you need to strive for balance by adding dimension to your hips. You're the woman who can wear hip pockets or a full or gathered skirt. You are also one of the few who can

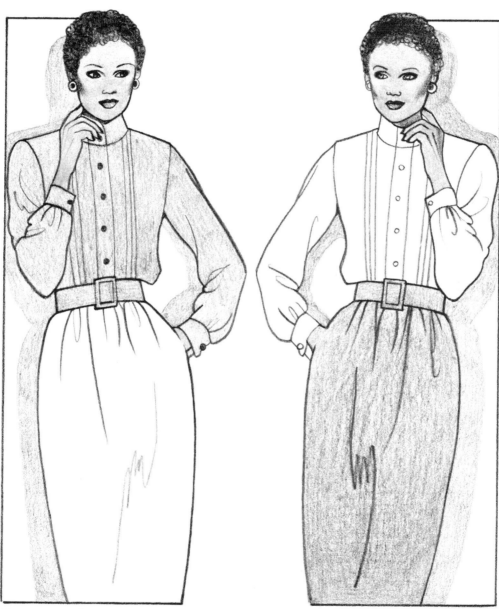

Short-waisted   Long-waisted wear a straight, box jacket, but you must balance this line with a pleated or flared skirt.

If your hips are too wide, avoid pockets or excessive fullness at the hipline. An A-line skirt works as long as it doesn't ride up, but an even better camouflage is a modified dirndl—not the lampshade you made in the ninth grade, but a very gentle gathering, about three inches more than the waistband, eased in evenly. Some slight fullness in skirt or dress is always good on you. But avoid cinching your waist. It's best to have fabric flow gently from waist to hips. Often a loose vest works well to camouflage a wide hip.

To flatter all hips, choose panties that give a smooth line to your garment. Bikini panties leave a ridge under slacks, unless you buy the kind with a wide lace band at the top. Smooth lines are youthful and sexy. The dent caused by bikini panties is not flattering. Bikinis are fine under loose garments. If you have trouble with a dent at the bottom of your panties, you may be buying them with leg bands that are too small.

If you need smoothing under slinky, revealing outfits, wear control-top panty hose or a whisper-weight panty girdle. A heavy girdle looks matronly and out-of-date and is not good for your circulatory system.

FANNY:
An ample derriere limits the number of styles you can wear, but it is a fairly easy figure problem to cover. Choose skirts with some fullness or an A-line, rather than a straight skirt. Be sure your pants fit properly, so they do not cup under the seat. The fit should be loose enough over your thighs to allow the fabric to flow smoothly from the fanny to the leg.

The style of your jacket is important, and a softly fitted jacket, moderately tapered, is always your best bet. A box jacket, with its straight lines, will not work with a large derriere, unless the jacket is short, above the crest of your fanny, and worn with a pleated or flared skirt. Avoid a box jacket altogether with pants. A tightly fitted jacket is equally unflattering, because it accentuates the curve of your fanny. Never wear a too-long jacket in an attempt to "cover up." The length of your jacket must be determined *from the front;* it should be proportional to your total height and the length of your legs (see "Legs" later in this chapter). A jacket that is too long for you only succeeds in making your legs look short and your body look top-heavy; you will ruin your total look. Instead, look proportioned and be sure your pants fit properly in back.

If your problem is a derriere that is too flat, you too need a skirt or dress with some fullness or a two-piece outfit that adds an extra layer of fabric where it counts. You may wear a tapered or box jacket, but a closely fitted jacket is too form-fitting. Why not let the taper of your jacket *suggest* what is (or isn't) really there?

If you have a flat derriere, one that droops, or a curved (sway) back, you will need to alter your pants and skirts by removing excess fabric from the waistline in back. A skirt that droops or cups in back is unflattering to any problem fanny.

One final note on the fanny: by the time you are thirty, gravity has usually worked its will and your fanny has dropped three inches or so. Check your shorts and tennis dresses for length in back as well as in front!

THIGHS:
Heavy thighs are common, but they also are the easiest figure flaw to disguise. Skirts and dresses with an A-line or slight fullness provide easy camouflage, as do pants that fit with ease over your thighs. Pants that are too tight call attention to your thighs, revealing their shape and size, whereas an inch of ease-

ment is slimming. Avoid pants that taper at the ankle, as this silhouette emphasizes the heavy thigh. The most flattering pants line is a slight flare or a straight leg with a hint of taper at the knee.

If the current trend in pants styles is not flattering to you, live out the season in skirts. Your best look will return another year.

LEGS:
If your legs are short, avoid cuffs on your pants; wear high heels to give the illusion of length; and keep your suit jackets relatively short—no lower than the crotch, and preferably at the break of your leg. Your blouses and over-tops should be even shorter than your suit jackets for a balanced look. Remember, you are aiming for overall proportion.

High-waisted styles are excellent for the woman with short legs, as they give the illusion of longer legs and height.

Although slightly long legs are an asset, too-long legs make it difficult to find clothes that fit and to achieve a well-proportioned look. Do wear pants with cuffs and wear jackets that end slightly below the crotch when viewed from the front. Avoid high-waisted styles in pants, skirts, and dresses (including wide belts). You are the woman who can successfully wear tunics, low-waisted styles (if your hips allow), and trim on your hemline.

If your legs are of average length, your best suit jacket length with *pants* is at the crotch. In years when hem lengths are just below the knee, a suit jacket worn with a *skirt* needs to be shorter in order to look proportioned.

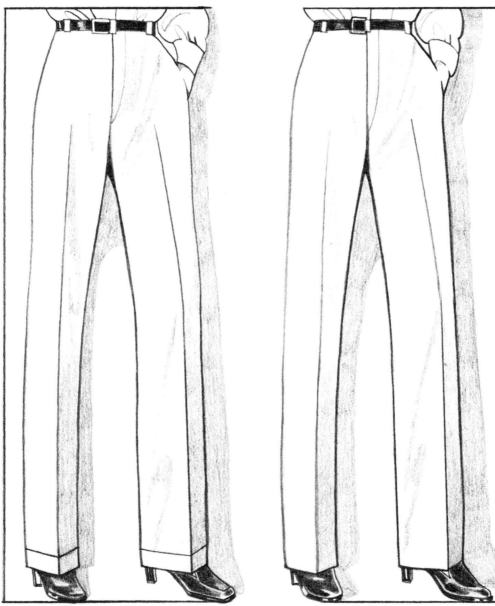

Cuff minimizes long legs.

For most of us a three-piece suit, consisting of pants, skirt, and jacket, is not a wise investment because the jacket will not be properly proportioned for both the pants and the skirt. The exception is the tall woman, or the one with long legs, because her skirt is automatically longer and is thus proportioned to go with a longer jacket. But during years when hemlines are lower, a three-piece suit will work because the proportion of the skirt is increased.

HEIGHT:

The taller and slimmer you are, the more styles you can wear. The tall woman can wear heavier fabric, more fullness, and low-waisted styles, if her figure permits. If you are quite tall, however, 5'7" or more, you will do best to avoid all high-waisted lines, including short, waist-length jackets and vests. These lines increase the illusion of height and sometimes make the very tall woman look too tiny on top, again ruining the proportion of her total body. Use a full-length mirror to make the final judgment.

By contrast, the short woman looks especially good in high-waisted clothes and shorter-length jackets and vests. A three-quarter sleeve, accessories or trim near the face, anything that draws the eye up, is good.

Attractive hem lengths are determined by your height as well as the shape of your leg. Midi-length hems shorten you and add weight, so wear longer skirts only if you really look attractive in them. A soft, floating fabric can be worn in a longer length than a heavy fabric. Looking in a full-length mirror, check the proportion of your hem to your size. Now look at your leg to see whether the hemline falls in a flattering place. (If you're wearing boots, you need only check proportion.) I use a piece of cardboard to determine flattering hem lengths on my clients. Hold the cardboard in front of yourself as you look in the mirror. Raise and lower it to see what happens to the shape of your leg. When you find a spot you like, have someone measure the distance from the floor. You can use this guideline for hemming all your skirts. Be sure you remember which shoes you are wearing, or, better yet, measure in stocking feet. Some women have slim, cylindrical calves and find that many lengths are flattering. But some of us have only one "good" spot and are best to stick to it, allowing fashion trends to change us only slightly.

WEIGHT:

The woman whose weight is normal can usually find lots of pretty clothes to suit her; she has to worry only about her special figure problems, if any. But if you are too thin or too heavy, you have a special need to create a *total* illusion, to enhance your overall look. In either case you should avoid clothes that are too tight and revealing; too-tight clothes accentuate both underweight and overweight bodies.

If you are extremely thin, you can soften the angles of your body and add dimension with some fullness in your sleeves and your basic silhouette, and by using prints and details. A simple tailored shirt on you is too plain, especially if you are tall. Give the eye more to look at by adding scallops to your collar, a large, special necklace or belt buckle, or perhaps interesting buttons or fabric texture. Just remember to scale prints, texture, bulk, and detail to your size; take care to be consistent with your clothing personality; and then have fun "adding" to yourself.

If your problem is overweight, the most slimming trick is wearing your colors. A color that flatters you draws the eye upward to your face and away from your body. Contrary to popular belief, black makes a body look larger. It is a heavy color and silhouettes your body against almost any background—a light wall, for example. If you are a Winter, black is fine because it flatters your face and draws the eye up. It is true that large prints increase apparent body size, but a solid, bright color—if it is *your* color—can be slimming because it diverts attention from your body to your total look.

Tent dresses are the worst possible line for the heavy woman. These dresses usually have only two seams and excess fullness, neither of which is slimming. The more vertical seams your outfit has, the slimmer you look, and often it is possible to shed ten pounds with your sewing machine by adding "fake" vertical seams. For example, I once bought a heavy denim skirt that stuck out like a tent and had only two side seams. The line was not flattering, so, without removing the waistband, I stitched a seam up the front and another up the back, taking a few inches of fullness out of the hemline and tapering to just a thread at the waistband. What a difference! We have done this in class for many clients, sometimes tapering a blouse, a skirt, or perhaps a whole dress.

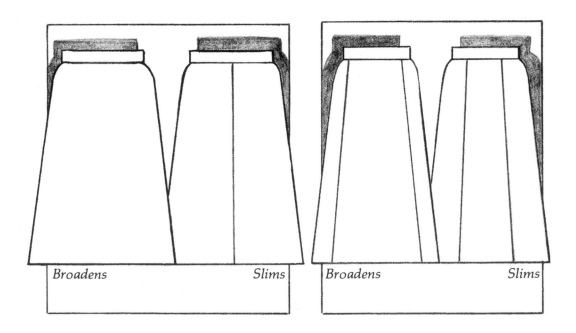

Broadens   *Slims*   *Broadens*   *Slims*

When your outfit has seams, panels, or gores, keep them close together for a slimming effect. A wide-paneled gore in a skirt or dress creates the illusion of a wide body, while a narrow panel makes you look slimmer. (The too-thin woman can use these same tricks in reverse to add weight.)

In general, the overweight woman looks best in a line that is cut with ease but not excess fullness, and a fabric that is slightly firm with a soft, but not clingy drape. Avoid bulky or stiff fabrics altogether.

If you dress carefully, people will see you as a whole, rather than zeroing in on your parts. Wear makeup, take care of your hair, and enjoy being pretty. There may be a diet and weight loss in your future, but meanwhile, dress to look great *now*.

CONCLUSION

Never worry about wearing the same line all the time, if that is the most flattering line for you. You can get variety through fabric, color, and detail. No one notices the line of your outfit if it looks good, but people invariably notice clothes that are unflattering.

Again, remember that any fashion is only as good as it looks on *you*. If you follow fashion trends to be "in," even when the current trend does not suit you, you are cheating yourself. But if you wear the latest fashion because it looks great on you, you've got the true fashion message.

And isn't it nice to know that while fashions and styles go in and out of vogue, you can go on looking your best year after year?

Color Me Beautiful

II
Put It All Together

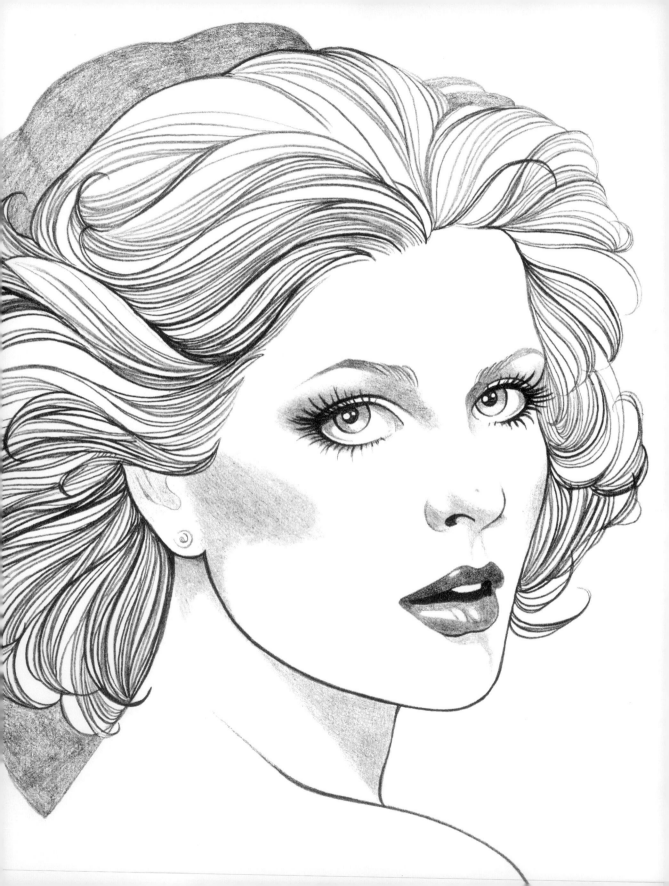

8

YOUR FACE :
Finding the Right Makeup

YOU HAVE YOUR COLORS, CUT OUT AND READY TO GO. YOU'VE explored your clothing personality to see how best to express your individuality. Now it's time to put it all together, starting at the top.

The right colors on your face are every bit as important as the right colors in your clothing. One is incomplete without the other. You will never look your prettiest in makeup that is alien to your natural skin tone.

Many women who attend my classes have found shopping for makeup a source of frustration, and they often appear at the first class in the wrong colors. How well I remember the times I was sent home with peach foundation to "match" my olive skin. What money I wasted on orange lipstick! Still ringing in my ears are the words of my aunt at that family reunion where I had wanted to look so good: "You certainly do get pale living in the East, don't you?"

Now that you know your season, the mystery of makeup is solved and it is easy to know what makeup colors are right for you. Whether for foundation, blush or lipstick, the principle remains the same. The warm seasons wear peach, orange, and brick red; the cools wear pinks, plums, and true reds.

Makeup consultants are often trained to match your makeup to your clothes. Happily, you are now matching your clothes to you. By matching your makeup to you, also, you will find that one set—foundation, blush, lip color, eye makeup—will blend with everything in your wardrobe.

Even if you prefer not to wear makeup, don't skip this chapter. After working with women of all ages and tastes for years, I am convinced that every woman looks better and wears her range of colors more attractively with a touch of color on her face. Some women need only a dash of blush or a hint of lip gloss, while others need more. Color, intelligently applied, maintains the glow of youth.

This chapter is primarily about color rather than technique. If you are inexperienced at applying makeup, take advantage of the free advice offered at every major department store. The people there are experts at applying makeup; you will be the expert on what color to apply. I have worked with many beauticians and, once they understand the palettes, they are delighted to learn about such a meaningful guideline to helping a client look her best. Our Color Me Beautiful Consultants also offer personalized instruction in application techniques as well as color selection.

As in all other aspects of fashion, beware of fads in makeup. Don't succumb to colors that don't look good on you. If brown tones are the rage but on you they don't fly, don't wear them. You can always be in style without sacrificing your best look.

SKIN CARE

Skin care is of course a must, and innumerable books already have been written on the subject. I will add only that in my years of study and consultations with dermatologists, both for myself and for my students, I have found two major fallacies in the method of skin care advocated by many cosmetics companies.

Fallacy No. 1: Everyone Should Wear Foundation. If you have clear, lovely skin that does not need smoothing, you do *not* need to wear a foundation. If you prefer no foundation, you can protect your skin by keeping it clean, sealing it with a toner, and moisturizing it if necessary.

Fallacy No. 2: Everyone Needs Moisturizer. Not true. If you have oily skin or skin that breaks out, it is harmful to put any cream on your face. A woman whose skin consistently breaks out should also avoid oil-base makeup—a water-base foundation is preferable. As you age, your skin will become drier, and eventually you will need moisturizer. Keep a watch on yourself, but don't be pushed into creams you don't need. Overmoisturizing can actually cause your skin to sag.

FOUNDATION

Foundation, or makeup base, derives from two basic tones: rose (cool) and yellow (warm). Winters and Summers wear foundations with a rose base, while Autumns and Springs wear those with a yellow base.

How do you tell the difference between a warm yellow beige and a cool rose beige? First, ask. Often the saleswoman knows her line well and is aware of yellow and rose bases. If she doesn't know, the name of the foundation can sometimes (though not always) be a clue. Yellow bases often are called "natural," "ivory," "peach," "golden," or "copper," while rose bases are typically called "rachel," "rose," or "sand." Some names give no clue to the tone of foundation. "Guadalupe Beige" is meaningless, so you will have to use your eye to judge.

Compare the beiges by putting a thick blob of each on your hand. A rose base will have a purplish or pink cast, whereas a yellow base will appear peach or yellow. You can see the tones when you are comparing shades. It's difficult to see tone in a color standing all by itself unless the shade is extreme.

A Summer usually has noticeable pink in her skin and needs a base that looks pink and blends with her jawline. Some Winters also fall into this category, and these women rarely have difficulty finding a foundation. Many Winters, however, have either white, beige, or olive skin, devoid of visible pink tones on the face. These women need to be especially careful to find a beige foundation with a *rose undertone.* When a Winter erroneously finds herself in "natural beige," she will look flat, perhaps a little sallow. If she ends up in peach, she will turn orange. Occasionally a Summer is sallow and needs to follow the same rule and avoid ending up in a yellow base.

If you are a Summer or Winter with a ruddy complexion, do not let a makeup consultant talk you into a yellow-base foundation in order to tone down your high coloring. Instead use a beige foundation that has no noticeable pink in it but that is derived from a rose base. This will tone down your ruddiness without detracting from your natural skin tone.

Depending on the depth of her coloring, the Autumn is best in ivory, peach, or copper tones. If she is just beige, she wears the "natural beiges" with yellow undertones. A sallow Autumn does best with a peach foundation, if she is careful that it blends with her jawline.

A Spring most often wears a light to dark peach foundation. She should avoid blue-pinks. Some Springs are pure ivory and are best in an ivory base, adding peach to the cheeks with a blusher. Ruddy Autumns and Springs can tone down their high coloring with a warm "natural" beige.

Some cosmetics lines are heavily weighted toward one base tone, and you may find nothing for you. Even the chemist who creates these colors is influenced by his or her own season, intuitively. Helena Rubinstein, before her death, was actively involved with the creation of her own line of cosmetics. She was a Winter. Now I know why I always had "good luck" at her counter. So if you aren't finding what you need, don't hesitate to say "none of these is right for me" and move on to the next counter.

Always check a foundation in natural light. Most stores have inadequate lighting, and what you see isn't what you get in the clear light of day. Test the shade of the foundation on your jawline. It should blend in perfectly when thinly applied. Never match foundation to your cheeks, as they have more color than the rest of your face. Makeup matched to cheek color will leave a line around the jaw.

Apply makeup thinly over clean skin that has been moisturized if necessary. Parched skin will absorb the foundation, giving you a heavily made-up look. Blemishes should be covered with a cover stick rather than a thick layer of makeup.

Do not spread makeup down your neck. Your neck is never the same color as your face, and no one likes to see fingermarks of color streaking down a lovely lady's neck. When blended perfectly to your jawline, the right color will not show and will serve the purpose of smoothing the face.

Once you've found a good base, you can order by phone (until the unhappy day it is discontinued). It will always be right for you and your clothing. With a summer tan, buy the same tone in a darker shade. Some women prefer to skip foundation in the summertime.

BLUSH

Blush gives eternal youth, and it can be applied so naturally that only you and your mirror will know. Winters and Summers should wear blushers in the rose family, ranging from blue-pink to burgundy. Some Winters may prefer a clear red. Autumns need blush in orange tones, preferably russet, terra-cotta, or tawny peach. They should avoid pink-looking peach. Springs must stay delicate and wear clear peach, coral, or warm pink, avoiding blue-pinks.

Creamy blushers work well for some dry skins, but powder blushers are easier to apply for a well-blended, natural look. Blush-on powders work well for all skin types and are especially good for oily skins. Gels are often difficult to apply, though the clear gel sticks are easy to manage and look extremely natural. They need to be reapplied periodically, as they tend to wear off.

Apply blusher along the cheekbone, beginning under the pupil of the eye and smoothing up into the hairline. Bring the color down the hairline slightly and back to the original point under the eye, forming a triangle. Do not bring blush lower than the bottom of your nose, in front, or into the circle area under the eye. Blend the edges for a natural look. Think of your face as a watercolor rather than an abstract painting. All color should be applied sparingly and blended smoothly.

But if you lack cheek color, be sure to use enough blush; it is possible to underdo it. If you have high coloring, you can use blush to reduce ruddiness, believe it or not. Nature seems to place cheek color all in front. It looks fine in the mirror because you see yourself only from the front,

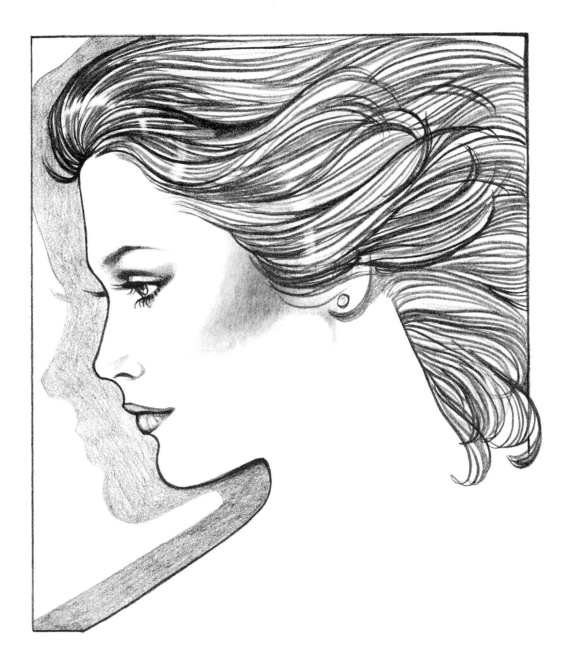

but others see you from the side. Add blush to the sides of your cheeks to complete the triangle. You will be amazed at how this little trick distributes the color, smoothing the cheek color into your face.

Soften your blush with age, as your skin lightens. Don't be a little old lady with two red dots on your face.

LIPSTICK

The same rules you used for foundation and blush apply to lipstick or lip gloss color: rose tones for the cool seasons, orange tones for the warm.

The intensity that is right for you depends on your age, the amount of color you have in your lips, how dark or fair you are, and your clothing personality. Use the printed color samples for your season as a guide when shopping for lipstick. Be sure to try out the lipstick testers on your lips rather than your hand, or you may be wasting your money. Very likely you will find one color that is just right for you and will go with your entire palette. A lipstick does not have to match your clothes, as long as it blends.

Winter is the only season who usually needs to own two tubes of lipstick, one to wear with the true red of her palette and the other for the rest of her clothes.

Winter is best in pinks, plums, burgundies, blue-reds, and clear reds, avoiding orange or yellow tones. If your skin tends to make a lipstick turn blue, try a frosted lipstick, which often alleviates this problem. Remember that Winter in general needs clear, rather than muted, colors. Some Winters need a bright lipstick, while others can afford to wear a subdued shade. Although a few look attractive in brownish plums and burgundies, most do not. The exception is the black Winter, whose reds and burgundies do need some brown in them. But even these colors must have life to them for the Winter woman to look her best.

Summer needs a softer lipstick than her Winter counterpart. Her pinks, while blue, will be best in light shades. She may also wear burgundy and plum tones and, if necessary, cheat into a warm pink to avoid becoming too blue. The brownish pinks and plums are okay if they are not too dark.

Autumns should look for brick red, orange, coral, peach, rust, mocha, and brownish shades. Some Autumns need bright colors, while others need a soft, subdued color. Autumns usually do not look good in highly frosted shades except for evening. They should avoid peaches that are too pink.

Spring may wear peach, warm pink, or coral. The pink should not be blue, and all of Spring's lipstick tones should be clear and not too dark. Some Springs do well in clear red, though most are better in softer tones. Spring is not the brown lipstick type.

In the summertime, or any time you have a tan, select a lipstick a shade darker, but in the same tone as the one you normally wear.

When applying lipstick, it is essential that you master the use of a lipstick brush or lip pencil. It is difficult to follow your natural lip line accurately with a tube, even a new one. Just outline the lip line and then fill in the rest with the tube. If using a brush, buy sable; less expensive ones will soon have little hairs sticking out in all directions. Begin at the center of your upper lip and follow the lip line to the left; then repeat from the center to the right. Do the same for the bottom lip. Never stroke all the way from left to right in one swoop, or your lips will be crooked.

I do not recommend using a contrasting color to outline lips unless you are striving for a theatrical rather than a natural look. If your lips already have a lot of color, you can use a lip pencil to outline your lips lightly and then blend the line with your finger. The pencil outline, blended, also gives added definition to your lips if you wear lip gloss rather than lipstick. It takes a little practice to outline your natural lip line, but it's worth it. The use of a lipstick brush or pencil elevates your total look from "almost" to "arrived."

EYE MAKEUP
Eyes are a beautiful, expressive part of a woman's face, and it is appropriate to accentuate their beauty. Yet many women make their worst errors in this effort. The object of eye shadow, for example, is to enhance the shape and color of your eye. You want people to say, "Look at the girl with the pretty blue eyes," rather than, "Look at the girl with the blue eye shadow!" *Never* let anyone tell you to make up your eyes to match your dress. That defeats the whole purpose of eye makeup.

Eyebrows:
Eyebrows should be plucked to follow the natural shape of the eye. Flat eyes usually are accompanied by flat eyebrows. Clean up the eyebrow area, but don't try to create a fake arch. Average to round eyes usually have arched eyebrows, and in that case plucking the arch area makes the brow attractive. Eyebrows growing toward the lid serve only to make the eye look smaller, so do pluck, but do it judiciously. Take a pencil and hold it against the outside of the nose and across the tear duct. The tip of the pencil will point to the place where your brow should begin. Now run the pencil from the nose to the crease at the outside of the eye to see where the brow should end. Pluck out the excess or feather in the missing area with an eyebrow pencil. Do not pluck brows so that they become too thin.

If you need an eyebrow pencil, choose a color based on your brow and hair color. Try it out on your forehead. Winters and Summers need charcoal,

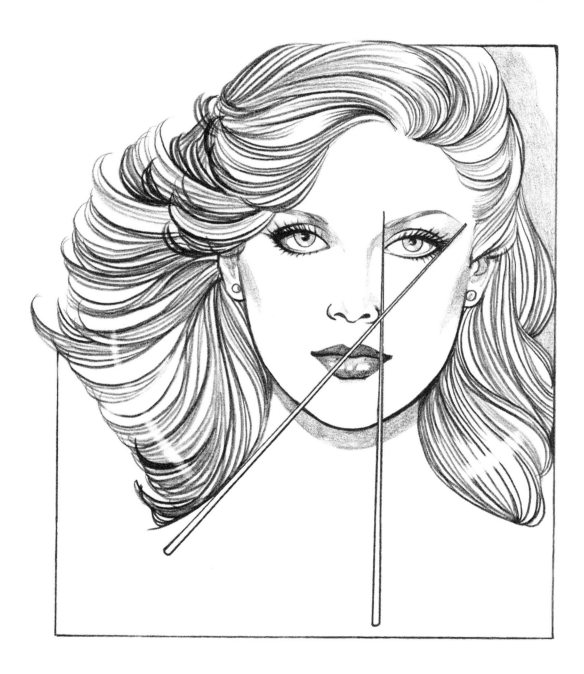

brown, or blonde tones that have absolutely no red in them (even if the hair has red highlights). They should look for grayish or taupe tones. Autumns and Springs are the opposite and should look for golden blonde, reddish brown, or dark brown eyebrow pencils.

Eye Shadows:
Eye shadows come in powders, creams, liquids, and crayons. Use whichever you personally find easiest to apply. I find powders the easiest to control. A matte finish is usually best as a highly frosted or iridescent powder will accentuate crepiness on dry or aging skin. If you prefer crayons, be sure you use a creamy one that spreads easily. You don't want to stretch the skin around your eye area.

Eyes are of three general types: deep-set (with little or no lid showing), average (with some lid showing), and prominent or sunken (with most of the lid showing). Eye shadows can bring out or recess certain eye areas. A light shadow brings out an area; a dark shadow makes it recede. Each eye needs to be treated individually, but here are some basic guidelines.

For purposes of illustration, we will divide the eye into three areas from top to bottom: the underbrow, the orbital bone, and the lid. Some women need a highlighter shadow on the underbrow, a second shadow on the orbital bone, and a third on the lid. Others have eyes that have room for only two shades, a pale highlighter on the underbrow and a color or darker neutral on the lid, brought slightly up onto the orbital bone.

Underbrow: A highlighter on the underbrow is a light neutral color that serves to open the eye and clarify the skin, eliminating pink or tired brown tones around the eye area. Applying the highlighter from the brow to the lid gives you a good, clear base for the whole eye area.

Lid: On the lid, it's best to use a color that blends with your own eye color, but in a considerably softer shade. It should either be the same color as your eye or a

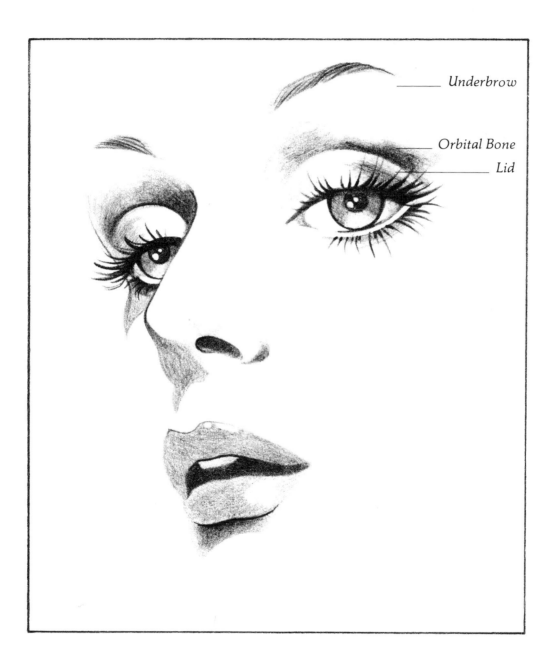

Underbrow

Orbital Bone

Lid

complimentary neutral. Be careful not to wear a shade that clashes with your eye color, such as blue shadow with green eyes. Golden brown eye shadows are good on many brown-eyed Autumns and Springs, while Winters and Summers must wear grayed brown tones such as taupe, mushroom, or cocoa. Brown-eyed Winters and Summers can also use smoked mauve, plum, or navy to bring out their eye color as these provide a complement to a cool brown eye.

A person with prominent lids must stick to neutrals, rather than colors, on the lid. These might be brown, gray, smoked navy, or smoked plum, depending on the person's season and eye color (see the charts that follow). Any color-color is glaring and calls attention to the lid rather than minimizing it. For such eyes, apply the highlighter in the crease and the dark neutral on the lid just near the lashes, leaving the rest of the lid as is.

For deep set eyes where no lid shows when the eye is open, use a very light shadow or highlighter on the lid. Any dark shadow will make the eye look smaller.

Orbital Bone: For most eyes, it's best to use a dark to medium neutral on the orbital bone. This neutral can also be brought down onto the other third of the eyelid to widen the eyes a bit. A deep-set eye is the exception; it is sometimes effective to bring the eye color rather than a neutral onto the bone area, lightly. Just a hint of muted color on the bone will bring out the color of the eye. If it is too bright, mix it with a neutral.

Choose the eye type in the accompanying illustrations that most closely resembles your own and follow the principles when applying your eye shadow.

Now use the following charts to find the correct basic eye makeup color for you. If your iris has two colors, you may use either. The lighter your skin, the lighter you apply everything. "Dark," "medium," and "light" mean relative to you. A brush is best for blending, but you can use a cotton ball or your fingertip. Remember, eye shadow means shadow, not bright color. Even color is used here to create a "shadow" effect for a natural look.

If you wear glasses all the time, you may apply eye makeup a little more heavily than other people, but be careful not to overdo it.

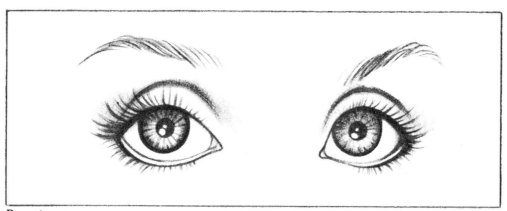

Prominent

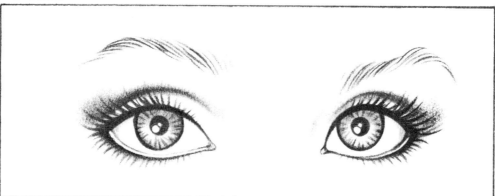

Average

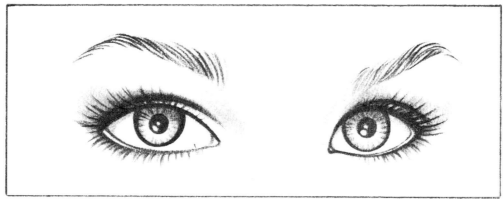

Deep Set

WINTER *Eyeshadow*

Eye Color	Brown	Brown-Green	Blue or Gray-Blue	Aqua-Blue	Green or Gray-Green
Underbrow (Highlighter)	Pale taupe/Gray	Pale taupe/Gray	Pale taupe/Gray	Pale taupe/Gray	Pale taupe/Gray
Orbital Bone and Outer Third of Lid	Gray, Smoked Plum, or Smoked Navy	Gray, Grayed Green, or Grayed Brown	Gray, Smoked Navy, or Smoked Plum	Gray, or Grayed Brown	Gray, Grayed Green, Smoked Plum, or Grayed Brown
Lid	Mauve, Plum, or Grayed Brown	Ash Green, Mauve, or Grayed Brown	Ash Blue, or Mauve	Smoked Teal, or Mauve	Ash Green, or Mauve

If you are extremely fair, you may wish to substitute off-white for pale taupe or gray highlighter under the brow. For the prominent eye, use smoked navy (which will appear gray when thinly applied) on the lid for brown and blue eyes, and gray or grayed green for green eyes. Above all, stick to cool colors with ash tones.

SUMMER *Eyeshadow*

Eye Color	Blue or Gray-Blue	Aqua-Blue	Green	Brown
Underbrow (Highlighter)	Off-White	Off-White	Off-White	Off-White
Orbital Bone and Outer Third of Lid	Gray, Grayed Brown, or Smoked Plum	Gray, or Grayed Brown	Gray, Grayed Brown, Smoked Plum or Grayed Green	Gray, Grayed Brown Smoked Plum, or, Smoked Navy
Lid	Ash Blue, or Mauve	Smoked Teal, or Mauve	Ash Green, Mauve	Mauve, Plum, or Taupe

Summers should not use dramatic eye makeup. Always blend well and keep subtle. For hazel eyes, pick the dominant color and use that column. For green eyes, use a gray-green shadow even if your eye has some gold in it. Avoid yellow-greens, as you are striving for cool tones. Many blue eyes blend with a smoked turquoise better than with an ash blue shadow. You can tell easily by applying an excess of each color, just to see which is better for you. Then blend. Occasionally a brown-eyed Summer will need smoked navy rather than mauve, plum tones on the lid, especially if her lid protrudes.

©Color Me Beautiful, Inc. 1984

AUTUMN *Eyeshadow*

Eye Color	Brown	Amber	Green	Blue
Underbrow (Highlighter)	Beige or Peach	Beige or Peach	Beige or Peach	Beige or Peach
Orbital Bone and Outer Third of Lid	Brown, Copper, or Muted green	Brown	Brown, or Muted Green	Brown, or Smoked Teal
Lid	Brown or Beige	Brown or Peach	Green	Smoked Teal, Brown, or Beige

For hazel eyes, choose the dominant color in your eye and use that column. For brown eyes, use golden or charcoal browns rather than red browns, which may make you look as if you've been crying. Beige is good on the deep-set lid. If you look tired in brown eye shadow, use a brownish green or subtle teal instead. Green-eyed Autumns can use their green color swatches for shopping. Find the green swatch that most closely blends with your eye and find an eye shadow that is a softer version of that color. Greens with yellow in them are best for you, but never select a bright green. Some Autumns can achieve a dramatic look in makeup quite successfully. But the more blonde and fair you are, the less makeup you should wear and the less dramatic should be your look.

SPRING *Eyeshadow*

Eye Color	Brown	Amber	Blue	Aqua	Green
Underbrow (Highlighter)	Ivory	Ivory	Ivory	Ivory	Ivory
Orbital Bone and Outer Third of Lid	Golden Brown, or Muted Green	Golden Brown or Peach	Brown or Smoked Blue or Teal	Brown or Smoked Teal	Brown or Muted Green
Lid	Brown	Brown or Peach	Blue or Smoked Teal	Smoked Teal or Soft Aqua	Green, or Golden Brown

Springs must apply eye shadow sparingly and blend it well. If you are extremely fair, rub most of it off with a brush or sponge applicator. Just a hint is enough for you. For hazel eyes, pick the dominant color in your eye and apply the appropriate column. Your browns should be soft and golden—subtle, not dramatic. For aqua eyes, use a smoked teal or aqua rather than a bright one. Some blue-eyed Springs are better in blue than in teal, see which blends the best with your eye. Green-eyed Springs look for yellow-greens rather than ash greens, but always soft and subtle.

Mascara:

Mascara is an excellent means of accentuating your lashes and toning down the eye shadow on your lid. It is best to use natural tones—blacks, browns, and blonde-browns rather than exotic colors. Again, you want to enhance your eye rather than call attention to your eyelashes. Apply mascara to your lower as well as upper lashes unless you have a protruding eye and wish to diminish its size.

Here are suggested mascara colors for each season:

Winter: Black (for extremely dark eyes only), brown-black, or brown, according to the depth of your coloring. Avoid red-browns.

Summer: Brown-black, charcoal, brown, whichever is closest to the color of your hair and eyebrows, but slightly darker. Avoid red tones.

Autumn: Brown-black, brown, whichever is best for you. Your mascara may have golden or red tones.

Spring: Brown, reddish brown, whichever blends best with your hair and brows.

False Eyelashes:

False eyelashes can be fun for the dramatic or romantic type woman. The most natural are the clusters that you apply individually. Use five or six clusters for each eye, applying short ones on the ends and medium-length ones in the middle positions. Many beauty shops will put these lashes on for you, though it is relatively easy to do yourself. These lashes stay on in the shower and last for a few weeks.

The strip styles look natural if the false lashes are thin, merely enhancing your own. These, too, should be shorter on the ends, longer in the middle. Lashes that are long at the outer edge will make your eyes look droopy.

Eyeliner:

Eyeliner is not for everyone. Many eyes, especially deep-set or average types, look smaller when eyeliner is applied to the upper lid. But with the advent of smudgy pencils or crayons the line can be softened with your fingertip to serve as a deep eye shadow. It is effective on deep-set and average eyes to use a touch of crayon on the outer third of the upper lid. Some brands of powder eye shadows can be used as liner when applied with a moistened eyeliner brush. The prominent eyelid needs eyeliner, in a neutral color, smudged along the upper lid close to the lashes. This helps make the eye recede.

All eyeliners should be a neutral or smoky version of your eye color—never a bright color. The exception is liner for the eye that is so deep-set that the lid does not show at all. In this case you may use a liner in the same color as the lid eye shadow, applied thinly at the base of the lashes, then blended with your finger or a brush. This color will barely show when the eye is open and will help bring out your eye color. The woman with deep-set eyes, as I mentioned previously, can bring her lid color lightly onto the orbital bone. Both of these techniques will "open" her eye and enhance her eye color.

All eyes except prominent ones can have the outer two-thirds of the lower lid underlined in a neutral color: gray or charcoal for Winters and Summers, brown tones for Autumns and Springs. Keep it thin, blend it with your fingertip, and then apply mascara.

CONCLUSION

With a little experimenting, you will soon find just the right lipstick, blush, eye makeup, and foundation for your coloring. All of it will fit in a pouch for easy

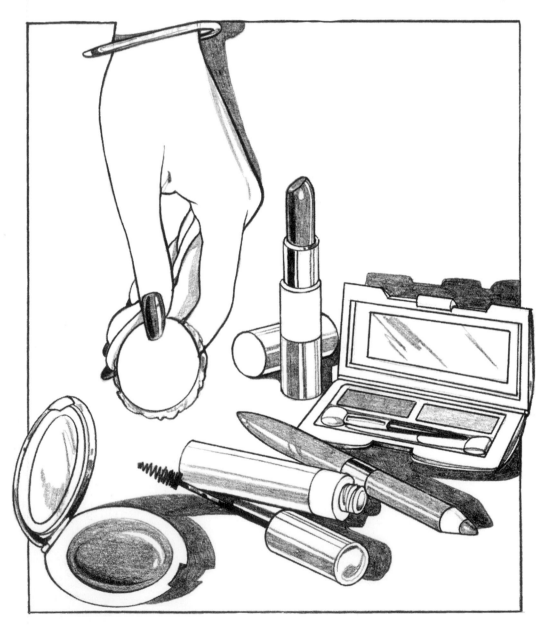

portability. In fact, with so little makeup you can afford to buy two sets, one for home and one for your purse.

These makeup guidelines are timeless. Whatever changes occur in the fashion world, you can retain your best look by adapting the fads or fashions to the color scheme of your face.

Makeup is an important element in putting yourself together. It need not be expensive, and it should be easy and fun now that you have the confidence to know what's right for you.

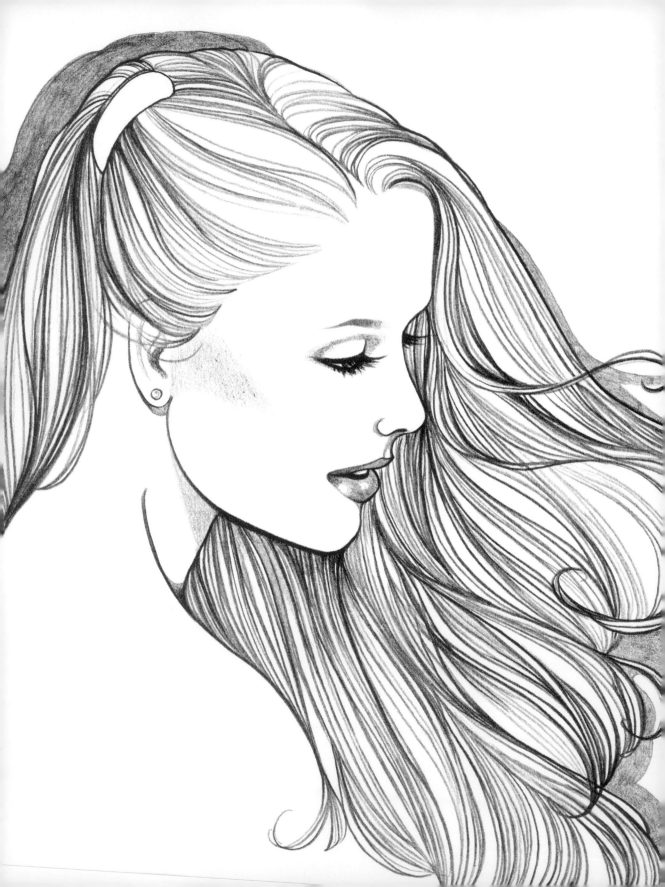

9

YOUR HAIR:
Getting the Color Right

HAIR COLOR

One of the first questions women ask me is "What color should my hair be?" It's a good question, since many women who dye or frost their hair are doing it in the wrong shade. In my classes I find that women want to color their hair for one of three reasons: to stay blonde, to cover gray, to give themselves a boost.

Nature usually does it right, and for many, doing nothing is best. But sometimes it is appropriate to color hair, and the secret to success is knowing what color to select. Hair color is simple once you know your season. To look terrific, any dye color, frosting, or highlighting should go *with* your coloring, not against it.

Of all the seasons, Summers most often feel drab and want to enliven their looks by doing something to their hair. Often they were blonde as children, and their hair turned mousy as they entered early adulthood. I recall one especially beautiful Summer who had been a towhead almost until her teens, and then her hair darkened. Instead of returning herself to her natural ash blonde color, she succumbed to the latest fad at the time, red henna. Her hairdresser convinced her that it was the very latest and that this change would give her the spiffy look she longed for. Henna on a Summer is harsh, aging, and unharmonious with everything about her. It clashes with her skin and her clothes. She must either wear the wrong makeup to go with the orange tone of her hair, or let her correct makeup clash with her hair. This beautiful Summer, who had not looked bad with her "mousy" blonde hair, now looked terrible. All she had needed were her colors. A Summer's face comes to life when she wears her palette, and her hair will look livelier, too.

Summers and Winters, the cool seasons, should always strive for ash tones in their hair. Autumns and Springs, with their warm skin tones, will look best in golden or reddish tones.

Winter: Most Winters have brown to black hair. Their hair is beautiful on them just the way it is. A Winter should *never* frost her hair, nor should she bleach it blonde or add red. It can look striking if it is totally white, but achieving that look through the bottle is usually less than exciting because it looks artificial. Best to wait until it turns white all by itself. A Winter can use natural or black henna, but never red. If you are a Winter, do not let your hairdresser talk you into highlighting, painting, or frosting. Your hair is likely to turn red if stripped with peroxide, and frosting succeeds only in making you look old.

The Winter woman's only question is what to do when she begins to gray. Winter is the season most likely to gray prematurely, and often the gray comes in attractively, creating a salt-and-pepper look. If you keep your hair short and chic, salt-and-pepper can be stunning. Long, unstylish gray hair is dumpy. If your personality does not thrive in gray hair, by all means color it, but insist on ash brown tones when covering gray. Your hairdresser (or you) should not mix ash brown with any color that has the word "warm" in it. "Warm" means that red will appear. Mix instead with ash blonde for a lighter, softer color. A Winter can also use a gray shampoo or one of the shampoo formulas that cover gray naturally. A little gray left in the hair serves to keep it soft in tone. Remember that as you age, your skin fades and it is wise to let your hair lighten also. The rare blonde Winter usually stays blonde and doesn't need to do a thing. Winter, be happy with yourself as nature made you. Spend your money on diamonds and leave your hair alone.

Summer: Summer's hair, whether blonde or brunette, often has a grayish cast that is beautiful with her Summer palette. The dark brunette Summer, like the Winter, should let her hair be. But a Summer who was once blonde or whose brown hair is light can be blonde successfully since she has a blonde complexion. Frosting is an excellent way for the Summer woman to add life and blondeness to her hair. She should strive for soft ash tones, avoiding all flaxen, golden, honey, or red tones, including henna. Some ash tones turn greenish, so she might ask her hairdresser to use a "warm ash" as long as it doesn't become too golden. The Summer often grays attractively and may wish to leave the gray for a naturally frosted look. If she wishes to cover it, she must use ash blonde or brown tones. Avoid all over-the-counter labels with the word "warm" as they usually imply a golden color. A few Summers have a reddish cast to their hair due to the intense red pigments in their skin. (Summer men often have ash blonde hair and red beards!) These Summers can use a gray shampoo to tone down the red if they wish or leave the highlights as they are.

Some Summers need contrast but want to be blonde. Ash blonde comes in many degrees, so don't forget the possiblity of dark ash blonde for facial contrast, with pale ash streaks or frosting for "glamour."

Autumn: The Autumn woman is the one who looks terrific in red highlights. An Autumn who was a blonde child and wishes to stay blonde should always use golden blonde tones. Ash blonde will make her pale and will not harmonize with her face and clothes. For the other Autumns, auburn, red, and warm brown tones are the best shades. They should avoid ash tones. Redheaded Autumns should never let their gray show until they are completely gray. As gray hair comes in on an Autumn, it tends to be yellow-gray—aging rather than chic. But once an Autumn's hair has turned completely gray, its overall warm tones can be most attractive. An Autumn is wisest to stay away from frosting. The two-tone look is usually not as flattering on her as highlighting or a painted effect, which looks like natural coloring from the sun.

Spring: Many Springs have warm blonde or brown hair that has darkened to a golden shade and looks beautiful just the way it is. If a blonde Spring wants to stay blonde, she should use flaxen or golden blonde hair coloring, never ash. She also should stay away from frosting, though she can use the painted or highlighting effect. A Spring is the youthful type and should not use any hair color that looks too sophisticated or appears gray. Her hair does not gray attractively, and she is wise to color it during its "coming in" years. But once it is completely gray, or white, its warm color is flattering. To cover gray, Spring can use auburn, golden brown, or golden blonde hair coloring. Some Springs are redheads and should keep that red hair forever. "Warm" is the word to look for on any bottle of dye.

To summarize:

Appropriate Hair Color

WINTER	SUMMER	AUTUMN	SPRING
Ash Brown	Ash Blonde	Golden Blonde	Flaxen Blonde
Blue-Black	Warm Ash Blonde	Golden Brown	Golden Blonde
If gray, her choice	Ash Brown	Red Brown	Golden Brown
	Frosting	Red	Red-Brown
	If gray, her choice	Strawberry	Strawberry
		Cover gray, unless hair is completely gray	Cover gray, unless hair is completely gray

HAIR STYLE

For hair style you should consider five points: your type, the shape of your face, the kind of hair you have, how handy you are with it, and your life style. A good hairdresser is your best friend, and you must give him or her as much information as possible about you and your hair. Discuss your facial shape and your life style. He or she is trained to help you achieve flattering lines. If your face is long and thin or rectangular, you will want to add fullness to the sides of your face. If it is round or square, you should minimize the sides. If you run into a stylist who wants to give you the "latest" without regard to how it looks on you, find another one. Don't hesitate to insist that you are the classic rather than the dramatic type if you are being urged to have a frizzy and you feel it isn't for you.

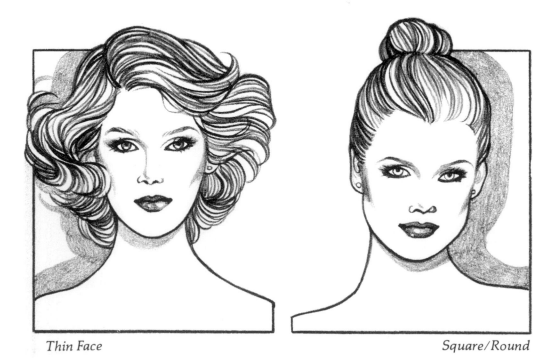

Thin Face   *Square/Round*

An excellent cut is a must. I have moved many times over the last fifteen years and one of my first problems after relocating is finding a good haircut. My best tip, tried and true, is to keep an eye out for someone whose hair looks the way you would like yours to look and ask who her hairdresser is. Most people, even strangers, are flattered to be asked and are happy to share this information. But remember that some hairdressers are best at cutting certain types of hair—naturally curly, limp and straight, thin or thick. For this reason it is best to find a woman whose hair is of similar texture to yours. Spend money on your haircut. A good cut makes all the difference in your daily appearance.

Long hair is fine for young women, but after thirty-five it is aging. Then it is best to keep shoulder length the limit, or wear a style swept off the face. After all, gravity tends to pull the face down, so we need to keep our hair on the "up" side. The older the woman, the shorter the hair. Many men love long hair, and I have had students in their middle years who keep long hair to please a husband or friend. Perhaps the reason is the youthful or sexual connotation of lengthy locks, but in both cases too-long hair defeats the purpose. Shorter hair on an older woman is both more youthful and sexier. Hair is a marvelous tool with which a woman can express her sexuality and how she feels about herself. Women who neglect their hair or wear an unflattering style are telling the world they are afraid to be beautiful.

Your hair style can date you, so do keep abreast of fashion. If you are wearing the same hair style you wore ten years ago, you undoubtedly look less youthful than you could. By the same token, wearing an "in," super-short, severe cut when you are a romantic needing femininity and curls is sacrificing your beauty to fashion. Be fashionable, be chic, but always be yourself. Adapt the current trend so that it works for you. The right hair color and style work wonders for your total appearance.

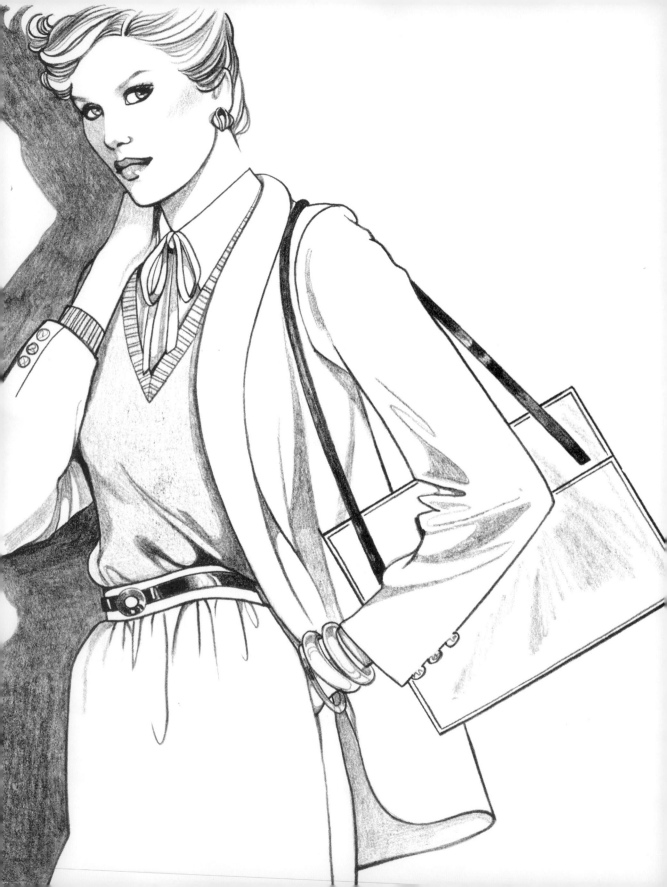

10

A WARDROBE THAT WORKS

HAVING A WARDROBE THAT WORKS IS EASIER THAN YOU THINK. Let your colors create it for you. With a plan and your palette you can have a coordinated wardrobe that will serve all your needs with fewer clothes, but more to wear. You will not have to ponder every purchase; you can rest assured that whatever you buy will blend with everything else in your wardrobe, thus saving you countless hours of shopping and countless dollars in "mistakes." The financial benefits of shopping from your palette are dramatic.

One client whom I had not seen for over a year called me during the holiday season to tell me how thrilled she was with the way her colors were working. "I just bought one skirt, and I gave myself seven new outfits," she said. The skirt was a print in a myriad of colors from her palette, and already in her closet at home were seven tops in several of the colors, ranging from a casual turtleneck to a dressy chiffon. The versatile cotton velveteen fabric of the skirt lent itself to dressing up or down. "I was shopping for several parties and thought I would have to spend much more to fill so many needs," she added. "I already have the right shoes, evening bag, and jewelry, according to my wardrobe plan. I can't believe how well my wardrobe is falling into place."

Because you undoubtedly have some colors in your closet that are not from your palette, your wardrobe will not be completely coordinated overnight. But if you stick to your colors from now on, you will gradually produce this miracle in your own closet. Phasing out wrong colors takes from two to five years, depending on what you currently own and how much you have to spend.

Make your old things work by mixing with a blouse, a scarf, or a vest from your palette. Don't buy anything new from a palette that is not yours. The full benefit comes once your entire wardrobe consists of only your colors.

The *approach* to planning a wardrobe is the same for every woman, whether she is a busy mother or an executive, has a limited pocketbook or money to burn, sews or lives in designer fashions:

1. Evaluate Your Life Style. Write down your usual routine over a normal two-week period. Add your evening activities and any hobbies or sports in which you participate. It takes only a few minutes to do this. Use your calendar to refresh your memory.

2. Start with Basic Clothes and Keep It Simple. A good wardrobe revolves around a few essential clothes in your season's neutral or basic colors. It's easy to add extras according to your needs. I like to keep my wardrobe relatively small. As soon as my closet starts to bulge, I know I've got clothes in there I'm not wearing.

To begin, let's look at the work potential of your palette. Each palette contains colors for every occasion. You have neutral colors, basic colors, and accent colors, colors for the beach, the bedroom, and the boardroom; colors for day and colors for evening; colors for wintertime and colors for summertime. You plan your wardrobe, year round, from your palette, choosing a color that is appropriate for that time of year.

Use the following chart as a planning guide:

	WINTER	*SUMMER*	*AUTUMN*	*SPRING*
Neutrals:	White	Soft White	Oyster White	Ivory, Cream
	Black	Rose-Beige	Beige	Clear Beige
	Navy	Rose-Brown	Camel	Camel, Tan
	Gray	Grayed Navy	Dark Brown	Golden Brown
	Taupe	Blue-Gray	Gold	Clear Gold
			Bronze	Warm Gray
			Olive	Light Clear
				Navy
Basic Colors:	Burgundy	Burgundy	Forest Green	Clear Red
	Blue-Red	Raspberry	Moss Green	Orange-Red
	True Red	Gray-Blue	Orange-Red	Coral
	True Blue	Deep Blue-	Bittersweet	Periwinkle
	True Green	Green	Red	Rust (for some
	Emerald	Blue-Red	Rust	Springs)
	Green	Watermelon		
	Pine Green			

Neutrals form the foundation of your wardrobe because they go with every-thing. Basic colors are the ones that are versatile and go with many others. Most are not too memorable and can be worn over and over again. Red, although bright, is a basic color, since it mixes well with neutrals and many other colors.

Choose your most flattering neutral or basic colors for your coat, suit, blazer, and basic dress, the clothes worn closest to your face. Any of your neutrals may be used for skirts and pants, shoes and bags. Generally, the darker neutrals are for wintertime, the lighter ones for summer.

The rest of your palette contains colors suitable for blouses, funwear, and accents. These are less versatile colors and are fine for extra dresses, skirts, or pants, but they must always be acquired *after* the basics.

Now let's discuss the most basic possible wardrobe. I call it a survival wardrobe. If you have one of each item listed, you have something to take you anywhere. Because this is a skeleton, it works for winter or summer clothes; simply adjust the fabric and sleeve lengths to suit hot or cold weather. We will add accessories to the plan later.

Your life style dictates how you expand or alter this basic wardrobe plan. The working woman should add another blazer, two additional skirts, several blouses, and one or two more versatile dresses, the kind that can go from day to evening with a change of accessories. The nonworking woman needs more pants and casual clothes. If parties play a big role in your life, add more cocktail clothes in several neutral or basic colors before adding one in a bright color. Some of my younger clients are students and say they have no need for cocktail clothes and never wear dresses. Eliminate what you don't need, but be careful. One dress is a minimum for almost any woman's wardrobe. You might, after all, get an unexpected invitation from someone exciting, and shopping in a rush often results in a compromise.

If your figure lends itself better to dresses than skirts, or to skirts than pants, simply substitute one for the other. A skirt and blouse ensemble often fills in for a dress. By the same token, a dress may be worn with a blazer to create the effect of a suit. Adjust according to your needs, keeping in mind that the first five items, plus a coat, are a must for any workable, ready-to-go wardrobe.

As you go through the list, make a check by each item that you feel is necessary to your life style. Right now, don't think about what you *have,* but consider what you *need.* Write a zero by the items that are unnecessary for you, and a number by the other items, estimating how many you think you should have. If your life style varies considerably from winter to summer, make two columns. Later you will go through your closet and see what you have and what is missing.

Last, add a section for special categories. If you are an avid golfer, tennis player, skier, or jogger, you will have special wardrobe needs.

Everyone needs a few hack-around clothes for painting the garage or digging in the garden. Most of us already have these, but do make sure yours are in your colors. You might as well be flattered in even your most casual attire.

Basic Survival Wardrobe

_____	Jacket	Your first suit jacket or blazer should be in a neutral, solid color from your palette with buttons to match. Keep the style simple for maximum versatility. Because this is the backbone of your wardrobe, the fabric and tailoring should be good. In the wintertime you might choose wool or ultrasuede and for warm weather, a linen, cotton, or silk blend.

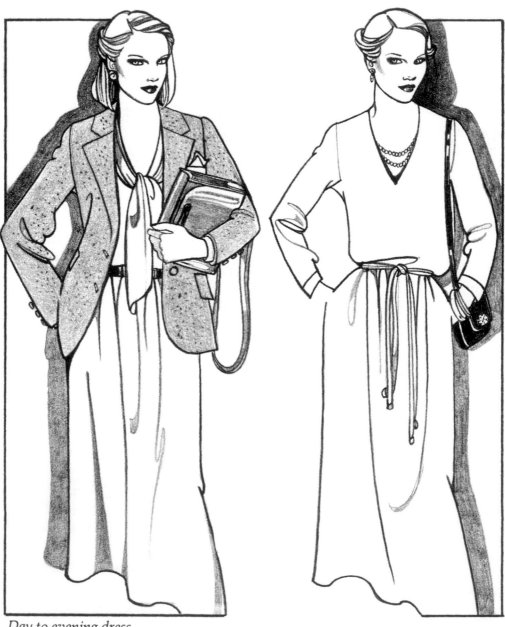

Day to evening dress

_____ Skirt
This skirt can be in the same color as the jacket or a contrasting neutral. It is best to keep it solid, but a tweed will work.

_____ Pants
The same rules apply to pants. A solid is more versatile for the first pair and is dressier than a tweed. These should be in a good fabric, wool for winter, cotton or linen-like fabric for summer.

_____ Dress
The first dress must be versatile, for daytime or evening. Keep the style simple, without a lot of trim or detail, and the color solid, in one of the neutrals or basics of your season. Wool blends, jerseys, cotton jerseys, and ultrasuede are good choices for wintertime, while jerseys, silk, silk-like blends, and cotton knits are flexible for summer or warmer climates. Once the first basic dress is acquired, you can add prints and more memorable colors.

_____ Blouse I
A tailored blouse in a solid neutral or basic color to go with your pants, skirt, and jacket is the first on your list. The fabric should be of silk-like polyester, silk, or jersey—something not too casual but not too dressy for work.

_____ Blouse II
This blouse can be more casual, in a print, plaid, or solid accent color, but in a less dressy fabric. It turns your jacket and pants or skirt ensemble into a suit that could go to a football game or any sports event, while still being appropriate for work or casual occasions.

_____	Dressy Blouse	A blouse in a shimmering, sheer or smooth fabric with dressy detail or a blousy cut turns your skirt or pants into a dressy outfit. This blouse should also be in a neutral or nonmemorable color, and can be worn with cocktail pants or a dressy cocktail skirt to further stretch your wardrobe.
_____	Sweater	A sweater in a basic color adds another dimension to your wardrobe. It goes with your suit (with skirt or pants), and as a separate with your basic skirt or pants, and with your jeans and casual clothes. Try a turtleneck or cowl (if a cowl suits you) for wintertime and a short-sleeved, cool knit for summertime.
_____	Cocktail Pants, Skirt, or Dress	Cocktail pants or skirts represent the most flexible approach to evening wear. Either should be in a basic color and a dressy, versatile fabric, such as a "silky" jersey, to go with your dressy blouse. You can add other tops, especially one in the same color as the skirt or pants, for maximum dressiness. A cocktail dress is fine, though it is not as versatile as separates. If you can have only one cocktail dress, it must be in a neutral or basic color. Your second purchase may be violet, fuchsia, or bright yellow-green—whatever strikes your fancy from your palette. It will be remembered and cannot be worn as often.
_____	Casual Pants or Skirt	This item can be of any casual material, from wool to denim, something comfortable that suits your life style. It can be more colorful, although, again,

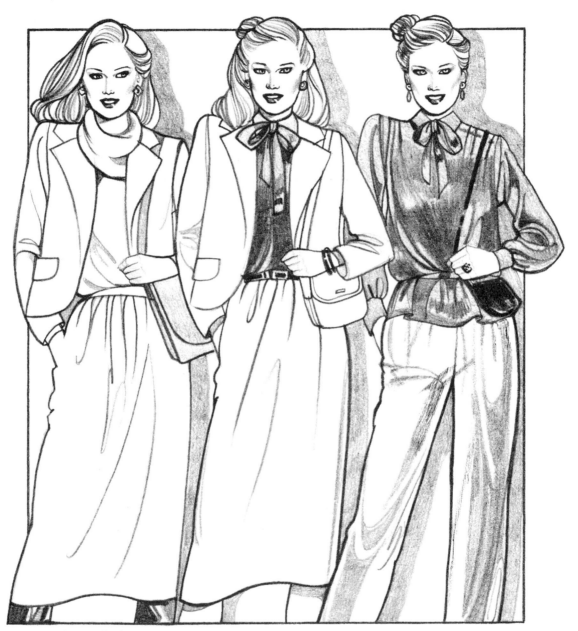

A versatile wardrobe

your *first* purchase should be relatively flexible. One outfit that falls in this category is pants with a top or "leisure jacket" to match. This combination is strictly casual and should not be confused with a pantsuit, which has a tailored jacket and can be dressed up to go almost anywhere.

_____ Casual
Shirt

Add a T-shirt, cotton blouse, jersey, turtleneck, or whatever you're comfortable in to go with your casual skirt or pants. Most people need to extend this skeleton plan beyond one of each in the casual department.

_____ Hack-
arounds

You need "old" jeans, cords, shorts, turtlenecks, T-shirts—whatever suits your fancy. Do toss out your wrong colors here. Hack-arounds are inexpensive and some people's life style calls for jeans most of the time. Don't cheat yourself out of looking good on a daily basis.

_____ Basic
Coat

In the wintertime, a basic coat for day to evening should be in a solid-color wool, with matching buttons, in a style that suits you, but is not too trendy. This coat is one of your major purchases, and you want it in a good quality and a style that is not quickly dated. A good, "classic" coat can last many years. Your basic survival wardrobe needs only this coat. You can add the following coats as your budget allows.

	Casual Coat	A casual coat is next on your list and can be a colorful wool, a trench coat, or even a leather coat. This coat should be fun, something to wear everyday. The working woman needs a trench coat, as it is businesslike, warm, and most useful in rainy climates. Others can wear a shiny slicker in a bright color to combat the rainy day.
	Jacket	Most of us also need some type of jacket, especially to wear with pants. This could be wool or even a parka, depending on where you live. If your money is tight, skip the jacket.
	Evening	Last, you will need something for evening. Your basic wool coat will do, but a velvet jacket or a fur (fake or real) would be your ultimate acquisition for a complete wardrobe. A fur is most flattering if it harmonizes with your hair. Although brown is not in the Winter's palette, she can wear brown fur if she is brunette. Both Winter and Summer should take care to avoid red tones in any fur, and women of these two seasons look lovely in white fur as well. Autumns can wear the red and red-brown furs. Spring is great in the creamy tone of beaver or in any golden brown or blonde fur. Use your swatches and your hair to guide your choice in fur.

In the summertime, or in warm climates, a light trench coat or perhaps just a suit jacket in a light-colored neutral will serve for daytime or casual evening, and for dressier occasions a pretty shawl is almost always appropriate.

———————— Special   Make a list here of your special clothing needs, the items you need for sports, hobbies, and so forth:

_____

_____

_____

_____

_____

_____

_____

_____

_____

_____

_____

_____

_____

_____

These items should fulfill your basic clothing needs. It isn't possible to anticipate every event, but as soon as you are able to have one of everything as a minimum, you will find that your wardrobe can handle most of the surprises that pop into your life.

On the following pages you will find suggested colors for your basic survival wardrobe. These suggestions are merely to show you how well your colors work together. Notice that your jacket goes with your pants, skirt, and dress, and your blouses go with everything. Substitute other colors from your palette, according to your preference and their availability during any given year. As you build on this skeleton plan, add more colors. Even one new blouse adds a new dimension to your wardrobe.

It makes sense to acquire first the things you need the most. Later, you can add that slinky at-home outfit you saw in the lingerie department, or some fad item you're dying to acquire. In a year or two, after you have a start, you will be able to add more fun things to your wardrobe.

Try to buy ahead of need. When you shop, keep an eye out for the items missing from your wardrobe, even though you may not need them right this minute. Then, when you do receive an invitation or an opportunity, you won't have to rush out to shop.

Remember, the purpose of your colors, aside from making you look your best, is to simplify your life. So let your plan and your palette deliver their promise, and you'll have a wardrobe that really works.

WINTER
Sample colors for basic survival wardrobe

	Wintertime	Summertime
Jacket	Black	White
Skirt	Gray	White
Pants	Black	Navy
Dress	Red	True Green
Blouse I	Icy Gray	True Red
Blouse II	Purple, White, and Black Paisley	Navy and White Stripe
Dressy Blouse	White	Purple
Sweater	Magenta	Navy (knit)
Cocktail Pants, Skirt, or Dress	Black	White
Casual Pants or Skirt	Navy	White
Casual Top	Red	Shocking Pink
Coat	Black	(above jacket)
Trench Coat	Taupe (Gray-Beige)	Icy Gray
Evening Wrap	Emerald Green (velvet)	White (shawl)

SUMMER
Sample colors for basic survival wardrobe

	Wintertime	Summertime
Jacket	Blue-Gray	Soft White
Skirt	Blue-Gray	Soft White
Pants	Soft White	Grayed Navy
Dress	Raspberry	Sky Blue
Blouse I	Gray-Blue	Blue-Green
Blouse II	Plum, Navy, and Rose Print on Soft White Background	Red, White, and Navy Print
Dressy Blouse	Mauve	Pastel Pink
Sweater	Blue-Red	Light Lemon Yellow
Cocktail Pants, Skirt, or Dress	Burgundy	Soft White
Casual Pants or Skirt	Cocoa	Gray-Blue
Casual Top	Deep Blue-Green	Watermelon
Coat	Grayed Navy	(above jacket)
Trench Coat	Rose Beige	Powder Blue
Evening Wrap	Burgundy (velvet)	Soft White (shawl)

AUTUMN

Sample colors for basic survival wardrobe

	Wintertime	Summertime
Jacket	Dark Chocolate Brown	Oyster White
Skirt	Coffee	Oyster White
Pants	Camel	Beige
Dress	Rust	Lime Green
Blouse I	Beige	Yellow-Gold
Blouse II	Teal, Camel, and Chocolate Brown Print	Orange-Red, Turquoise, and Beige Stripe
Dressy Blouse	Beige	Salmon
Sweater	Bittersweet Red	Bright Yellow-Green (knit)
Cocktail Pants, Skirt, or Dress	Dark Chocolate Brown	Beige
Casual Pants or Skirt	Forest Green	Camel
Casual Top	Jade	Orange
Coat	Dark Chocolate Brown	(above jacket)
Trench Coat	Beige	Beige
Evening Wrap	Dark Chocolate Brown (velvet)	Beige (shawl)

SPRING
Sample colors for basic survival wardrobe

	Wintertime	Summertime
Jacket	Ivory (or Soft White)	Light Warm Beige
Skirt	Ivory	Light Warm Beige
Pants	Camel	Light Clear Navy
Dress	Red	Peach
Blouse I	Clear Salmon	Light Periwinkle Blue
Blouse II	Orange-Red, Camel, Ivory Print	Bright Coral, Golden Yellow, and Navy in Tiny Floral Print
Dressy Blouse	Light Warm Beige	Warm Pastel Pink
Sweater	Golden Brown	Yellow-Green
Cocktail Pants, Skirt, or Dress	Light Warm Beige	Ivory
Casual Pants or Skirt	Golden Tan	Buff
Casual Top	Dark Periwinkle Blue	Light Clear Gold
Coat	Golden Brown	(above jacket)
Trench Coat	Light Warm Beige	Ivory
Evening Wrap	Ivory	Soft White (shawl)

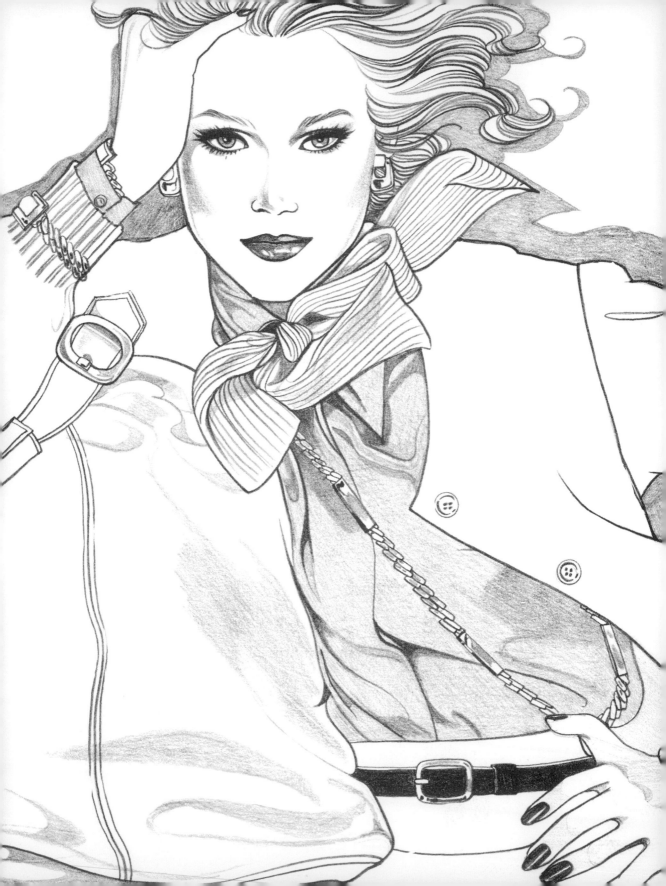

11

ACCENT ON ACCESSORIES

ACCESSORIES PROVIDE A FUN AND INEXPENSIVE WAY TO CREATE excitement in your wardrobe. If you have avoided them because you didn't think you knew how to choose them, your packet of color swatches will now be your personal fashion consultant. You can hardly go wrong when buying shoes, bags, jewelry, scarves, or belts, because your palette is so compatible.

SHOES

Shoes should generally be in a neutral that blends with the color of your skirt or pants. A contrasting neutral is fine as long as the color value is similar to the hemline of your skirt, dress, or pants—usually darker, is best. In the summertime or in a warm climate, you may go lighter or use the white or bone from your season. Bright shoe colors must be repeated somewhere else on your body, preferably near your face. If you wear red shoes with a blue outfit, for example, wear a red scarf.

Build your shoe wardrobe on neutrals, then add the colors. In any given season you will find two or three neutral colors that will work with anything in your wardrobe. In wintertime, your choices might be as follows:

Winter	*Summer*	*Autumn*	*Spring*
Black	Navy	Dark Brown	Medium Brown
Navy	Gray	Tan	Tan
Burgundy	Rose-Brown	Olive	Navy

In summertime and warm climates, choose the following:

Winter	*Summer*	*Autumn*	*Spring*
White	Off-White	Bone (Yellow)	Off-White
Black	Bone (Rose)	Tan	Tan
Bone (Taupe)	Navy	Brown	Navy

Isn't it comforting to know that you *need* only two or three shoe colors? An Autumn has no need for navy; a Winter no need for brown. Of course, you may add shoes ad infinitum, if shoes are your thing; but most of us appreciate being free to spend our money on an extra outfit.

STOCKINGS

Four pairs of stockings or pantyhose in a neutral skin color keep you in stockings at all times. When one runs, buy another. Buy your hose in the same color. When one leg of your pantyhose runs, cut it off and save the top and the good leg. You can wear two one-legged pantyhose at the same time, since the panties are thin enough to be comfortable when worn together. If you have two "partials" of the same leg, turn one leg inside out.

The tone of your neutral stockings should be based on your season. Winters and Summers want gray-beiges or rose-beiges. Autumns and Springs wear golden beiges. Even your stockings reflect the totality of your look.

Dark or textured hose call attention to your legs and should never be worn if your legs are heavy. It is a fallacy that dark stockings are slimming! Only if you have very good-looking legs can you wear colored stockings successfully. If you do wear them, use neutrals from your palette, of course.

BAGS

For everyday wear, you can have one basic handbag for wintertime and one for summer. The Winter does well with a dark gray bag, as it goes with black or navy shoes. Summer can use gray-navy; Autumn, medium brown; and Spring, tan.

Your bag should be in a neutral, either the same color as your shoes or lighter. It does not have to match the shoe, but it must blend. In general, it is best to draw the eye upward by having dark colors at the bottom (shoes) and lighter or brighter colors as you move up your body (bags, scarves). Accessorizing upward adds height, slims, and highlights your face.

In the summertime, Winters and Summers can use a white straw basket-weave, and Autumns and Springs a straw-colored bag, which will go with everything and take you anywhere.

For evening at all times of the year, Winters and Summers use a little silver envelope to go with all their cool colors, and the warm Autumns and Springs carry a gold bag (you'll see why after you read about jewelry). Remember to keep your personality in mind when choosing bags and shoes. Both the size and the type should relate to you.

JEWELRY

Here is your chance to make a personal statement. Your choice of jewelry reflects your type and your personality. We have already discussed the appropriate styles and shapes of your jewelry when we explored your clothing personality.

The metals in your jewelry are most important. White metals harmonize with the cool Winter and Summer colors, while gold tones harmonize with the warm colors of Autumn and Spring. You may be unhappy about that, but if you hold a piece of silver and gold jewelry against each of the palettes, you will see immediately which looks better. Notice how beautifully the silver tone blends with the Winter and Summer palettes? Now place gold against these palettes. You must admit, it clashes! Repeat the test by holding the gold against the Autumn and Spring colors: harmonious, luxurious, and right. Now the silver; it clashes.

The best jewelry for Winter is silver, platinum, and white gold; pearls with a white or gray cast; white ivory; and white coral. And Winters look beautiful in diamonds! Summer uses the same white metals but may add rose gold, rose pearls (the expensive ones) and rose ivory. Autumns may wear any gold, brass, or copper tones, wooden jewelry, and tortoise shell. They can wear cream-colored pearls. Springs also need gold metals but must be careful to keep the color and design delicate. Usually copper and brass are too bold for them. They are also best in creamy pearls.

You may wear any stones that blend with your colors. Use your swatches as a guide and set the stone in the metal of your season. The same is true for costume or enameled jewelry. Your colors are a guide for everything!

If you are young, you can begin collecting jewelry in the metals of your season, including your wedding ring! Many of us already have jewelry that's "not ours," however. As a Winter, I solve this problem by wearing my gold jewelry with the colors from my palette that are closest to the colors of the warm palettes: white, taupe, royal blue, and true red. You can do the same by wearing your "off" jewelry with those of your colors that are close to colors from an "opposite" season. It is possible to have your jeweler plate yellow gold with white gold and vice versa.

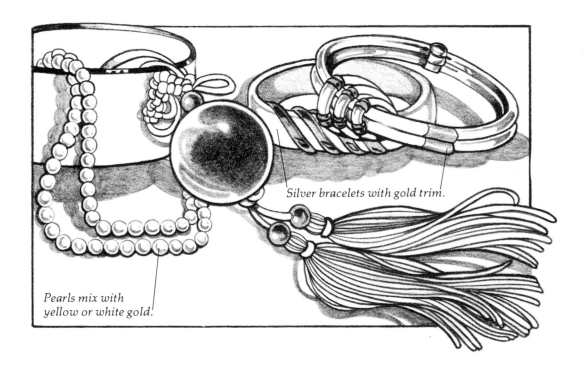

Silver bracelets with gold trim.

Pearls mix with yellow or white gold.

Yellow gold has a luxurious look that is hard to replace with a white metal; but mixing yellow gold with a white metal can give you the rich look you want without clashing with your palette. For example, you can mix metals in chains, bracelets, and two-color earrings. For Summers and Winters, pearls are another answer. I wear pearl earrings as a basic, because they give a dressier and more elegant look than silver. Pearls can also mix with either white or gold metals. For a sportier look, silver is great. Autumns and Springs can achieve almost any look, from dressy to casual, with gold.

Buy earrings first, chains and necklaces second, a bracelet third, a ring fourth, and a pin last. Start with earrings because they are what really make you look "dressed." In class, I keep some simple earrings on hand to demonstrate the effectiveness of this one accessory. A client is transformed from plain to chic with the snap of a metal clasp. Generally, an Autumn or Spring does well with a medium gold hoop or a button—smooth, brushed, or "twisted." A Winter or Summer can have a silver hoop, a button, or a large pearl. Brushed metal is versatile because it can be sporty or dressy, while shiny metal is casual unless the style is quite elaborate.

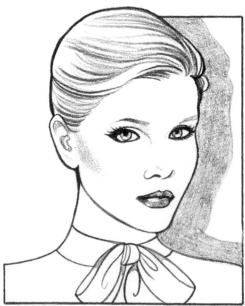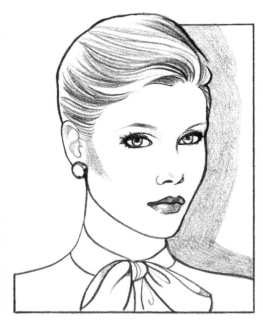

Earrings add the finishing touch

Jewelry is best organized into groups. With a wardrobe of basics, you can use your jewelry and scarves to dress an outfit up or down. Plan three groupings of compatible jewelry: one casual, one dressier, and one formal. These can often be worn with the same dress. Simply change jewelry at five o'clock and you're set for an evening out. Here is a sample of groupings:

Casual (Shiny)	*Dressier* (Brushed)	*Formal* (Sparkly)
Shiny earrings in silver or gold	Brushed metal or pearl earrings	Earrings in pearls or a stone for your season
Informal pin or casual necklace	Brushed metal pin	Pin or necklace with pearls or stone
Simple bracelet	Dressy bracelet or ring	Bracelet with stones; pearls; ring with stones

Be sure to add any missing jewelry items to your wish list. Although it takes time to acquire jewelry, it is exciting to keep it in mind as something to look forward to. Husbands, friends, and family will appreciate knowing that their jewelry gifts are not only meaningful but also really suit you.

Try to keep any trim on your shoes or bags in the metal of your season. Often a shoe repair shop can replace one buckle with another. Sometimes, however, it isn't possible to find the right "hardware," so choose a bag or shoe with minimal trim.

Always replace buttons with others of the right metal or color for your season. That's easy.

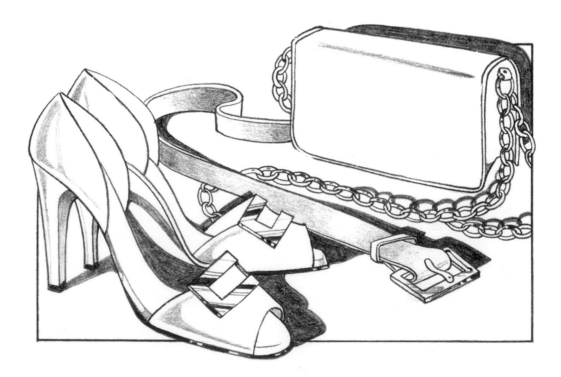

SCARVES

Scarves are a vital part of your wardrobe; they are your means of bringing the right color to your face while you are phasing the wrong colors out of your wardrobe.

The secret to wearing a scarf happily is securing it to your garment in strategic places with *straight pins,* angled so that they won't stick you. A safety pin is difficult to fasten, and by the time you've struggled with it the scarf is pinned crooked.

Scarves are one of my favorite accessories. Even if you have a short neck, you can wear one, as long as you keep the fabric soft so it is not too bulky. A scarf can turn you into a fashion plate and add infinite variety to your wardrobe. A basic silk dress can go from morning to cocktails simply by clever scarf accessorizing. Try a long, striped, multicolored cotton (yes, cotton can mix with silk) sashed around your waist or twisted and knotted around your neck for a colorful, casual look, and switch to a soft, printed silk and dressier jewelry for evening.

A scarf can be draped in a thousand ways, and anything you invent goes if you wear it with confidence and secure it with a straight pin (unless it's around your neck, of course). Any other pins are strictly for ornamentation. Here are five effective ways to tie a scarf:

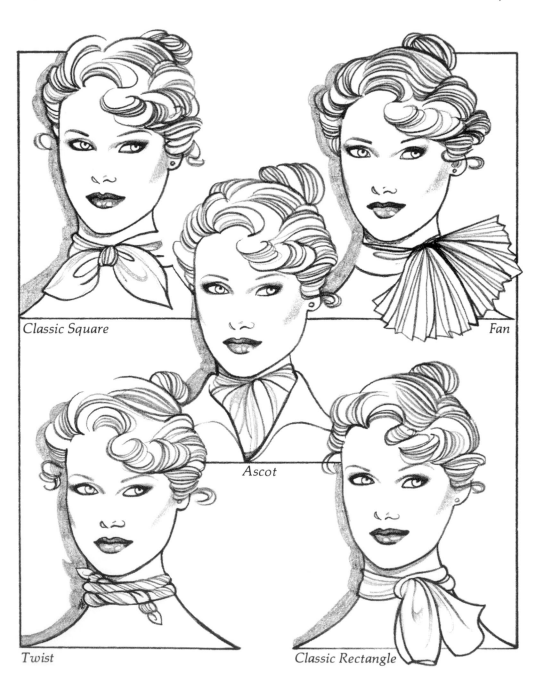

Classic Square

Fan

Ascot

Twist

Classic Rectangle

Classic Rectangle

Fold a long, skinny scarf lengthwise until you have a band. Fold it in half, wrap it around your neck, and insert the ends through the loop formed by the fold. Pull taut and secure with a pin, rather than a knot. Arrange in front or off to the side.

Ascot

Open a square scarf (large or small) and grasp the center. Tie a knot right in the center. Turn it inside out so that the knot is underneath. Take two opposite corners around your neck and tie in back. Tuck the front into your collar and pin it to your bra.

Fan

Take a large square scarf and fold it back and forth until the entire scarf is pleated into one narrow strip. Holding the ends so the pleating won't fall apart, wrap the scarf around your neck and tie once in front. Do not knot, but secure with a straight pin or a stick pin. You have two fluffy fans, which may be centered or flared to both sides or off to one side. This is a spectacular feminine touch, a dynamite addition to any basic outfit.

The Twist

This technique requires a long rectangle and looks best if the scarf has a print, stripes, or multicolors, though it can be a bright solid. Knot both ends of the scarf near the edges. Twist and twist until the entire length of the scarf is a twisted rope. Keep it tightly twisted while wrapping it around your neck twice, bringing the ends to the front. Rather than tying them, tuck the ends into the rope, lapping them over and under until you have created an abstract "knot." This scarf trick is for the dramatic or tall, sporty type, and it does require a medium to long neck, but it's great fun if you can wear it.

Classic Square

Fold a square scarf on the bias and tie it with a knot around the neck, with the tails in front or off to the side.

SECOND LAYER ... AND A THIRD

Adding the extra interest of a vest or jerkin or sweater is an inexpensive way to put zest into your whole look. Be sure to choose a fabric and style that suit your personality and figure. A loose vest can smooth the hipline and camouflage bulges. How about a vest in a shimmery fabric to give your evening pants or skirt yet another versatile twist? In wintertime, a long-sleeved sweater with a scoop or V neck over a solid or print blouse can really spruce up an otherwise plain skirt and blouse ensemble. Or try a blouse over a blouse, one tucked in, the other as a jacket. You can even add a third layer with a belt, tie, or sash if your figure permits.

HATS

Hats go in and out of fashion, and they're fun, if you are comfortable wearing them. Keep the color lighter than or the same color as your neckline.

When you try on a hat, stand in front of a full-length mirror; don't sit behind a table. Only then can you see its proportion in relation to your height and size. Don't forget to check the hat from the sides and back to see whether the shape is flattering.

A hat can increase or decrease the apparent size of your head if your head is small or large in relation to your body. Make these adjustments in the size of the brim, rather than the crown. The crown must fit your head accurately to look just right, but the brim may be any size as long as it is not wider than your shoulders. A tall woman can wear a larger hat than a short one.

If you live where the winters are cold, pick a warm hat that goes with the coat or jacket you wear most of the time.

GLOVES

Since gloves are no longer mandatory for the "well-groomed" look, you may not want to own any, other than a warm pair for winter. But if you do want a stand-by pair, your best choice is three-quarter-length kid gloves in the white or bone of your season. They can be crushed to wrist length and worn with any sleeve length.

If gloves regain their popularity, look in an etiquette book for proper lengths to suit the occasion. Always keep gloves in a light neutral from your palette. Your hands move, and they are not the best place for a bright accent color, except for outdoor sportswear.

Your warm winter gloves should be in a neutral to match or blend with your coat.

NAILS

If you wear colored nail polish, your nails become an accessory, too. Color calls attention to your hands, so stick to clear or buff if your hands or nails aren't your best asset. Otherwise, choose a nail color that blends with your lipstick. It can be lighter or darker as long as it blends.

BELTS

A belt is a great way to add interest to an outfit. If you have a wispy waist, you can show it off with a wide belt or one of a contrasting color. Otherwise, stick to narrow belts in neutral colors. A skinny belt in the metal of your season is a wonderful addition to your wardrobe. I consider it a basic, unless your waist says no. Even a large waist can have a belt buckle peeking out from a vest.

GLASSES

The frame of your glasses should be in the metal of your season, or in a color that harmonizes with your hair. As with fur colors, brown plastic frames are appropriate for a brunette Winter, even though brown is not in her palette. Again, Winters and Summers avoid red-brown tones.

The shape of your glasses should softly follow the shape of your face, but should not emphasize a pronounced facial contour. For example, if your jaw is square, your glasses should be squarish with rounded edges, rather than sharply squared. Proportion the size to your face, and keep the width of your glasses the same as your temples. Watch that your glasses do not go too far down your cheeks, or your face will look "droopy." It is best if the top of your frame is even with your eyebrows or a bit higher. If you can, take a friend when you shop for glasses, since it's pretty difficult to see yourself without the lenses.

If you want tinted lenses, choose a 5 or 10 percent tint the same color as your eyes, unless you are a brown-eyed Winter or Summer. Like brown eye shadow, brown lenses may give these seasons a tired look. Brown-eyed Winters look great in mauve and brown-eyed Summers in rose, and these will look best with your clothes, too.

Sunglasses do not need to be as basic and can be in a metal, neutral, or any fun color from your palette. If they are prescription sunglasses, you will probably want them in a neutral frame to go with all your summertime wardrobe.

CONCLUSION

Once you're dressed, stand back and take a good look in your full-length mirror. Do you need more, or less, or is your outfit just right? Accessories should be balanced, and no one accessory should be so bold that it detracts from your total look. Many women, however, are more likely to avoid accessories than to go overboard, for fear of looking overdone. Certainly, it's possible to go too far. One woman bedecked in too many pins and bracelets is enough to scare anyone away from accessories permanently. Everyone knows the rule: "When in doubt, don't." However, this is your opportunity to be creative, so take a risk and *do*. But whatever you do, do it with confidence. Accessorizing takes practice, trial and error. Have the courage to try a new look.

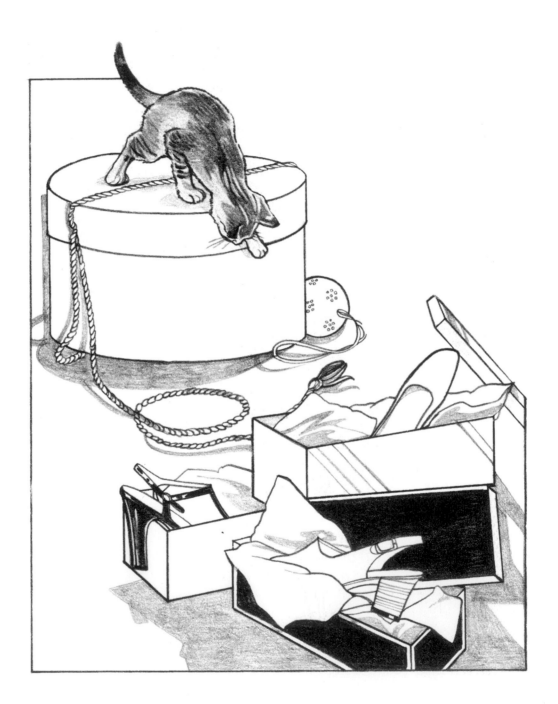

12

UNCLUTTERING YOUR CLOSET

NOW THAT YOU KNOW WHAT TO LOOK FOR, LET'S GO THROUGH your closet. Most of us are attached to our clothes, and it is hard to see them objectively. Ask yourself whether each garment in question still plays an active role in your wardrobe.

Allow time. You will never again have to spend this much energy on your wardrobe. From now on it will be much easier, so console yourself with that.

Four wardrobe problems crop up frequently.

Most common is simple accumulation of clothes, one outfit at a time, by the woman who buys for events as they occur. Her closet contains a shirt here, a pair of shoes there. Each was purchased to go with something now discarded, and it currently matches nothing. This closet is a mix but not a match.

Then there is the closet containing too many clothes. This woman buys impulsively, never gets rid of anything, and has decision confusion when it is time to get dressed or go shopping.

A third problem is common to the woman whose weight fluctuates. She has three wardrobes, each in a different size, so she has both too many and too few clothes.

Last is the problem of too few clothes, either because the woman has financial limitations, or because she is depriving herself (feeling guilty or waiting to lose weight), or because she feels insecure about what to buy, or because her life style centers around blue jeans.

The first step in solving any wardrobe problem is to organize your closet, so you can see what you have and what you need. The following guidelines will help you get uncluttered, as well as show you how to incorporate your season's colors into your existing wardrobe, while phasing out "wrong" colors as you can.

One

Remove everything in your closet that is not your current size.   We are going to dress the body you have now. Even if you are left with three garments, that's all you have to wear anyway, so there is no point in making yourself miserable by staring at clothes that don't fit. Put the too-big or too-small clothes in another closet or in the attic, keeping only the ones that are still in style and are your color. Stop waiting to buy clothes until you've lost weight. Look as good as you possibly can *right now*.

Two

Remove everything in your closet that you haven't worn for a year. I have consistently found that an item unworn for a whole year will not be worn this year either. The only exception might be an evening gown, because you haven't been invited to a formal party. Be ruthless. You are not doing yourself a favor having idle clothes taking up space in your closet. For each item, ask yourself: Is it your color? Your type? A good style? If you haven't worn it lately, think of three good reasons for keeping it. Otherwise, take it to the thrift shop where it can start doing someone else some good.

Three

Separate your right colors from your wrong colors, setting aside the wrong ones for the moment. Organize all your right-color clothing in groups, putting similar items together: jackets, skirts, pants, tops, dresses, and so forth. If possible, line up your shoes and handbags so everything in your closet is in sight. Now add the wrong-color clothes that you feel are necessary to your wardrobe for now.

Any clothes in your wrong colors that you really don't love or need are best discarded. Often you can trade clothes with friends of other seasons. I gave my beautiful, expensive beige coat to a favorite Autumn friend, and when she weeded out her closet she gave me a marvelous black leather purse.

If you have too many clothes at this point, weed out excess duplicates. Twenty shirts are more than anyone needs. So are too many dresses, suits, or skirts, for that matter, regardless of how expensive or beautiful they are. It is of no advantage to either your closet or your peace of mind to have an overwhelming number of clothes. I always suggest to the woman with too much that she create a skeleton wardrobe out of her favorite clothes, then add some extras and take a good, hard look at everything else.

Four

Make yourself a wardrobe chart to post in your closet. I am including my favorite charts for you to hang there right now if you want, though you may need to make larger ones to give yourself more space for each category. One is for your wintertime clothes and the other for summertime.

Fill in the chart that is appropriate for the current time of year, saving the other for later. Begin with the basics from your correct colors—jacket, skirt, pants, dress. Then, in parentheses, add the clothes from your wrong colors, ones you feel are still good. The parentheses indicate to you that you will eventually want to replace these items.

The chart is designed so that you can mentally dress yourself. As you list your basic clothes at the left, you can write in the appropriate shoes, handbag, scarf, or belt in the corresponding column at the right. Use a smaller version to plan your wardrobe for travel.

I like to number my shoes so I don't have to keep writing "navy heels." If some of your accessories are wrong for your season, keep only those that are essential during your transition period. Any stray shoes, bags, and especially scarves in the wrong colors should be given away. It is a blissful feeling to part with the last of the clothes that are not the true you. Then you are on the road to beautiful simplicity.

Underwear is included to remind you of special needs for those outfits that require a low-cut bra, a black slip, or whatever. I added that column after I had the experience of being on vacation with a brand new sheer dress and a half-slip that was ten inches too short. I searched all over vacationland for a full-length white full slip and couldn't find one. I had to buy a camisole for the top and a floor-length half-slip that I cut off with some borrowed scissors. I thought about a slip the day I bought the dress, but I forgot about it while packing.

Sample Chart

Wintertime Wardrobe		Shoes	Bag	Scarves	Belts/ Hats	Under- Wear
Jackets	BLACK (SUIT) NAVY BLAZER		(1) BLACK (2) NAVY		Burgundy HAT	
Skirts	GRAY WOOL BLACK WOOL (SUIT) NAVY GRAY TWEED	(1) BLACK High (2) NAVY			BLACK BELT	
Pants	BLACK GRAY TWEED	(3) BLACK LOW HEEL				
Blouses and Sweaters	White Magenta NAVY WHITE			BLUE: RED PAISLEY Burgundy PRINT		
Vests	NAVY					
Dresses	BLUE Ultrasuede BLACK Wool RED Wool	(2) (1) (1) or (2)	(2) (1) (1) or (2)			
Cocktail	BLACK pants, top ICE GRAY DRESS PURPLE SILK Dress	(4) Black, dress (5) Silver (4) or (5)	Silverbag " "			BLACK low cut Bra Sandlefoot . Stockings
Casual: Dresses	Burgundy velour Red corduroy	(1) or (3) (3)				
Skirts	Denim wool plaid	(6) Navy low-heel (3)				
Pants	Jeans	(6)				
Tops	Red turtleneck Green " Black Sweater			Challis print		
Coats	BLACK WOOL TAUPE LEATHER FUR JACKET					

On the following pages are blank charts for you to fill out.

Wintertime Wardrobe	Shoes	Bag	Scarves	Belts/ Hats	Under- Wear
Jackets					
Skirts					
Pants					
Blouses and Sweaters					
Vests					
Dresses					
Cocktail					
Casual:					
Dresses					
Skirts					
Pants					
Tops					
Coats					

Summertime Wardrobe	Shoes	Bag	Scarves	Belts/ Hats	Under- Wear
Jackets					
Skirts					
Pants					
Blouses and Sweaters					
Vests					
Dresses					
Cocktail					
Casual: Dresses					
Skirts					
Pants					
Tops					
Coats					

Five

Make a list of the items missing from your wardrobe. After you see what's missing, arrange your list in order of priority, putting what you need most at the top. For example, you may find that while you don't have a perfect basic— a solid-color, simple-style neutral—you may have something that will serve the purpose. Perhaps you have a houndstooth jacket instead of a solid, but it is giving you the suit you need for now.

This year a coat might be your priority. Because a coat is a major purchase, it may be the only thing you buy until next season except for a few accessories. Or you may feel you can wear your coat, even if it is the wrong color, and put your money into a jacket or dress. You must decide according to your needs and life style.

Your priority shopping list can be tucked into your purse with your colors so it is handy when you go shopping. If you know you need a basic dress to complete your wardrobe, you can keep an eye out for it while shopping for other things. Don't forget to list the jewelry you want. You are buying in advance of need, which is sensible rather than impulsive. We all know it's never there when we really have to have it.

Six

"Carry your wardrobe with you." In our wardrobe classes at Color Me Beautiful, the final accomplishment is "having your wardrobe on a safety pin"! Here is the way we do it. Cut a three-by-five card into thirds. Then clip a bit of fabric from the seam allowance of each garment in your wardrobe and glue it to the card. If the fabric would unravel, write the color on the card. Put your jackets on one card, pants on one or two, then skirts, dresses, and so forth. Now assemble your cards on a safety pin, and you have your entire wardrobe to take shopping with you. Sometimes it's hard to remember the fellows back home, especially when deciding on tops or scarves. Your packet of colors and your safety pin take the guesswork out of all your purchases.

With your wardrobe in order, you can begin to build sensibly. Updating a wardrobe from year to year is relatively simple. Perhaps you will add a vest, a skinny overbelt, and a blouson dress or blouse to bring your last year's clothes up-to-date. Often it takes only an accessory, a silk flower, or one item in a "new" fabric to keep you in style.

An uncluttered closet and an overview of your clothing needs give you direction for shopping and for spending your money wisely. At the same time, with a little yearly weeding and updating, you will have a well-coordinated, easy-to-care-for wardrobe forever.

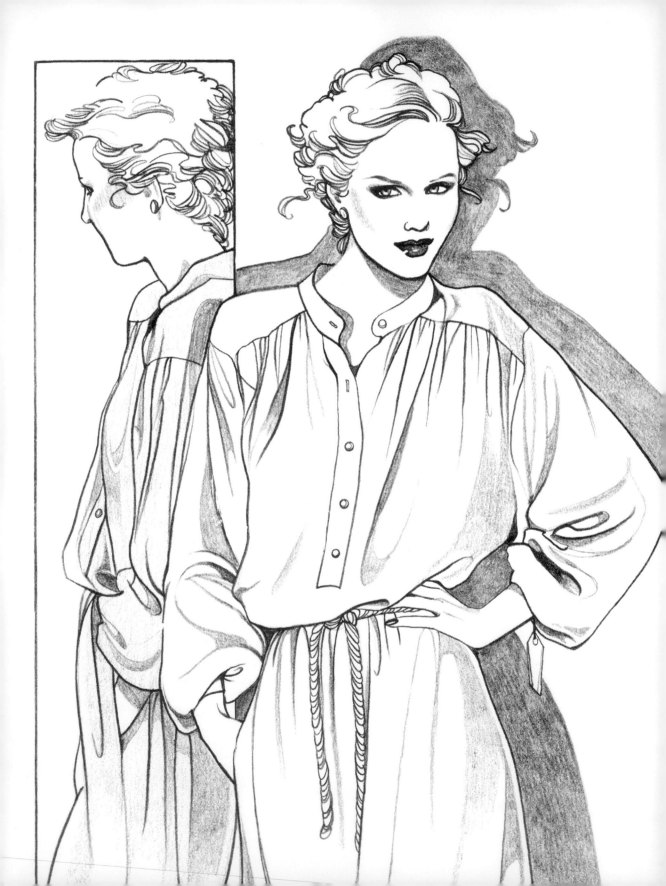

13

SHOPPING SANELY

BEFORE I HAD MY COLORS, I SPENT FIVE YEARS TRYING TO BUY A wool pantsuit. After living in California all my life, I was suddenly confronted with winters in cold New York, and pantsuits were coming into vogue at the time. The first fall, I tried on everything in my size, but nothing seemed to look good and, after all, a good pantsuit is expensive. The next fall I tried again, traipsing from store to store; and so it went, year after year. Finally I had my colors, but now I also had a three-year-old in nursery school. Any young mother knows that nursery school gives you two hours in which to accomplish all shopping, the alternative being shopping with a tired child. Armed with my packet of colors, I entered my favorite department store, cased the sportswear department, and in twenty minutes had pulled everything available in my size and colors—a total of five outfits. Only five, because it was fall and the racks were full of the usual fall colors. The third try-on was it—stunning—though the jacket needed minor alteration for a perfect fit. What a change! The culmination of a five-year hunt had taken an hour and a half, leaving me just enough time to make my nursery school pickup. I spent money on that purchase, but I knew it was right and wore the suit for years.

To shop with my colors as a guide is a pleasure. No wonder I had never found satisfactory clothing for myself in the fall. Never realizing that color was the factor, I had blamed it all on style and fit, the bulkiness of fall fabric, the terrible "new" designs, the ten pounds I had gained. Fall is no longer intimidating. Now that I accept the fact that most years fall clothes will not feature my Winter colors, my eye looks only at what's for me and there is always something nice.

Here are some shopping "Do's" and Don'ts" to help you save time and make your shopping decisions easy and rewarding.

Do: Shop with your colors, and look only *at items in your colors.*

Be sure you understand your colors. Familiarize yourself thoroughly with your palette and the color concept of your season.

Always shop with your swatches. The eye cannot retain a color image for more than a few seconds. It is difficult to tell whether that hot pink dress hanging on the rack is Spring's, Summer's, or Winter's, unless you have another pink for comparison. Put your swatch right up against the garment and, if necessary, take both to a doorway for better light. Often store lighting distorts color. Remember, you have some color territories in which you can shop freely, using your swatches as a guide. But a few colors in each season must be matched as closely as possible if you are to look your best.

You will find that your own season will usually be the best time of year for shopping, as that is when your colors are most often presented. During the other three seasons, you will have less from which to choose, but as your eye becomes accustomed to spotting your colors, you will find enough. One terrific outfit in your color is far more valuable than two in the wrong colors.

Occasionally, a fashion trend will be in your favor, enhancing your color selection during your "off" seasons. But some years will be better than others, so it is vital for you to build your basic wardrobe to carry you over a lean year. When designers are pushing muted shades, Winters and Springs will have to ferret out the few clear colors available. And that's the year for Autumns and Summers to stock up. When clear and bright is fashionable, Winters and Springs can buy for the future.

Long-sleeved blouses in year-round fabrics can be bought off season. I rarely wear long sleeves in the summertime because I live in a hot, sticky climate; but whenever I see a long-sleeved blouse in a color that would be suitable for my wardrobe, I buy it. It may not be available in the fall when I need it, because fall usually means earth tones.

Autumns and Summers have the easiest shopping year round; Winters and Springs must do more hunting. It's a small price to pay when the reward is guaranteed compliments and guaranteed good feelings about yourself. Besides, you will find that shopping is much faster now. Even if there is nothing for you, you will spend only a few minutes scanning the racks. You still have your money, your time, and your energy to check out another department.

You can take advantage of sales, knowing that whatever you buy at the end of this year's season will go with the unknowns you will buy next year. But remember your colors. A sale item is a bargain only if it looks good on you. A two-dollar scarf is a two-dollar waste if it doesn't flatter.

If you have a figure problem—be it weight, extra long legs, or a chesty bosom—I strongly advise finding yourself a good tailor or dressmaker. Shopping for fabric in your colors is easier than finding ready-made clothing in special cuts and sizes. Many of my overweight friends say that they are lucky just to find something that fits, so a dressmaker is a frugal and morale-boosting investment. (I consider it a waste of money to buy anything unflattering.) Being heavy doesn't mean you can't be pretty.

One of my Spring students uses a dressmaker for her winter clothes because it is hard to find the delicate Spring colors in winterweight fabric. She has a small but exquisite wardrobe and insists that it costs no more to have clothes made than to buy them in better department stores, and they are far less expensive than designer clothes. Springs should not overlook the soft white that appears in wool blazers, slacks, and suits during the cold winter months. This white is so versatile that everyone can wear it!

Do: Be aware of the fashion industry's color cycles. Be open-minded about which of your colors you will buy.

Shopping with a specific color in mind may lead to frustration and disappointment. The fashion industry pushes specific colors each season, and these, along with certain standard colors, are virtually the only colors available. If you are determined to buy a navy blue coat in a year when brown, gray, and burgundy are the fashion colors, you will only disappoint yourself. First see which colors in your palette are popular this year. Then choose the most flattering.

Understanding the fashion industry and its cycles is a great help in achieving your best look year after year. Buy your colors when you see them. Choose a classic style that will last and *build* a wardrobe.

Even though it is sometimes frustrating to cope with planned obsolescence and unpredictable hemlines, change is exciting, and we can appreciate the creative talent of designers who devote their time and energy to our clothes. And by pushing only a few colors each season, manufacturers can coordinate accessories—shoes, bags, jewelry—to complement the year's fashions. Imagine how confusing it would be if every color were available all the time. The stores would pop their seams, and you would have a nervous breakdown sorting through the merchandise. Industry must offer selective colors, and it's a favor to the shopper, too.

We who know our colors do not have to worry about planned obsolescence. This year's shoes will go with next year's clothes because all our colors go with each other. Build that wardrobe and you stay in control, no matter what the fashion world is offering.

Do: Learn to say "no."

When you walk into a store, you are bombarded with merchandise, all saying "Buy me." By buying only colors from your palette, you impose a pleasant discipline on yourself. Rejoice in knowing what *not* to look at.

People can't hoodwink you into buying unflattering clothes unless you let them. When a salesperson says, "This is the very latest; everyone is wearing it," resist. You are not everyone—you are you. Buy fashion only if it really looks good on you. You can always be in style in your own special way.

Remember you have a perfect right to shop and try on as many garments as you like. The sales personnel are being paid to help you. They are already receiving compensation, so you do not owe them a purchase. How many of us have succumbed to sales pressure, buying something and returning it later when a different salesperson was on duty? I did. But no more. Your colors can give you the confidence to say yes or *no*.

Do: Find a salesperson who is your season.

People automatically like their own colors—salespeople included. Unless they are trained in color, they will invariably show you the clothes that look good on them. Even when I hand a salesperson a packet of colors for myself or a client, I find that unless she is the same season, she will inevitably waste our time showing us innumerable wrong colors. Even though you show her your green, she will bring you clothes in her green. Find a salesperson who is your season, and she will become your shopping ally. She's the one who can run around finding you that red blouse because she knows where all the merchandise is hidden. Make use of salespeople. Most really do enjoy helping you, especially when they know what you want!

Men tend to use sales personnel more than women. They are always in a hurry to get in and out of a store and are often happy to have a salesperson "show" them what to buy to ease the decision-making process. It is essential for a man to have a salesperson of his season. On one shopping expedition, an Autumn salesman was helping my husband and me (my husband is a Summer). We asked to see blue suits, and the salesman kept showing us brown suits. My husband tired after five minutes—his usual shopping span—and began muttering "let's go" while angling toward the exit. Hanging on to his shirttail so he couldn't escape, I was scanning the racks myself, knowing we had not seen all the merchandise. Our discouraged salesman wandered off, and along came another salesman, a Summer who whipped out a number of gray and blue suits, one of which we bought five minutes later. My husband's agonies are over, as his favorite Summer salesman does well for him every time.

I have been hired by department stores to train their salespeople, and the experience has proved that their new awareness of color does make them more valuable to customers. Many stores, however, have not yet trained their salespeople to be color sensitive. So, until that happy day arrives, choose your helper by coloring rather than by personality.

Buyers also dramatically influence the selections in any given store, so pay attention to the merchandise you generally see in the store as a whole. It may or may not be for you, depending on the season of the buyer. My Autumn friend finds everything she needs at a particular boutique where I consistently find nothing. Once I met the owner, who is also the buyer, I saw why. An Autumn, of course.

Don't: Shop with a friend unless she (or he) understands your season.

Shopping with a friend can sometimes be a hindrance to your best look because, unless she has her colors too and understands that you and she may be different seasons, she, like the salesperson, will intuitively steer you into styles and colors that are suitable for her, not you. Your colors are your best guides when you shop.

If you want the fun of shopping with a friend, be sure she understands your new colors. Spend some time discussing both of your types and personalities. Give her the test in Chapter 4 so she'll have her colors, too. Then you'll really be able to help each other.

Your favorite man has color prejudices too, so be careful. He may love brown tweed and urge you to buy it without being completely aware of its suitability for *you*. If you're a Winter, and he wants you in tweed, show him you care in salt-and-pepper tweed or houndstooth—the look he likes, but the color that's right for you. He'll be convinced the moment he sees how great you look.

Don't: Buy implusively.

When shopping, work toward completing your basic wardrobe. Buy first the clothes you need most, using your priority list as a guide. If you see a dress you like, but you already have enough dresses, don't buy. Many of us accumulate the clothes we find easiest to buy for ourselves and consequently never reserve enough in our budget to buy something else we really need. If you have trouble finding pants that fit, and you need pants, resist that extra dress and keep hunting. On the other hand, when you see an item that is missing from your wardrobe, grab it, if your budget allows. This purchase is not impulsive. It's part of your plan.

Do: Spend the most money on the clothes you wear the most.

Invest your money in the clothes that really count. If you wear a suit only occasionally, it's fine to buy a less expensive suit and put your money somewhere else. But if you wear a suit to work everyday, you need quality. It would be a mistake to squander your budget on an expensive cocktail dress for one occasion, if it means skimping on a suit. The suit must be of a good cut and fabric to hold its shape wearing after wearing. A lesser-quality garment in this case would be a poor investment, costing you more money in the long run because it would have to be replaced so quickly. Invest in the suit and hunt for less expensive evening attire.

Do: Be well groomed when you shop.

Dressing well when you shop gives you two advantages: You will be better able to judge clothes on yourself, and you will receive better service. It isn't fair, but it is true that salespeople will respond to you according to the way you look. If you wear dungarees and your gardening shirt when you shop for a nice dress, the salespeople will assume that you are a person with limited taste and/or no money to spend and they will concentrate on the woman who looks as if she will buy. Dressed carefully, I have often walked away with only a scarf, but much attention and solicitation from a fawning salesperson. Another time, dressed in my hack-arounds, I have practically had to force someone to take my money for a rather expensive purchase.

You can best judge how a garment looks on you if you are wearing the right underwear, stockings, and shoes. If you are shopping for jeans, wear pants; but if you are looking for a dress, suit, or evening gown, dress accordingly. It is impossible to decide whether an elegant evening dress is flattering in your sneakers.

Do: Develop a shopping routine.

Shopping by color is the biggest timesaver in the world! It is a boon for the working woman or anyone who requires a complete wardrobe but whose life style leaves little time for shopping. First find your size. Then pull the items in your color. Third, check out the personality of each outfit—is it your type? Next, look at the style and cut of the garment. Now, feel the fabric; scrunch it to see if it wrinkles. Is it appropriate for the intended occasion and for your needs? Check the laundering instructions. Labels give instruction on care, and it is disappointing to discover at home that the "wash-and-wear" skirt you bought has to be dry-cleaned. Now try on the garment and check for fit. Don't overlook the possibility of alterations. Although color works magic, a poor fit is still noticeable and detracts from your best look.

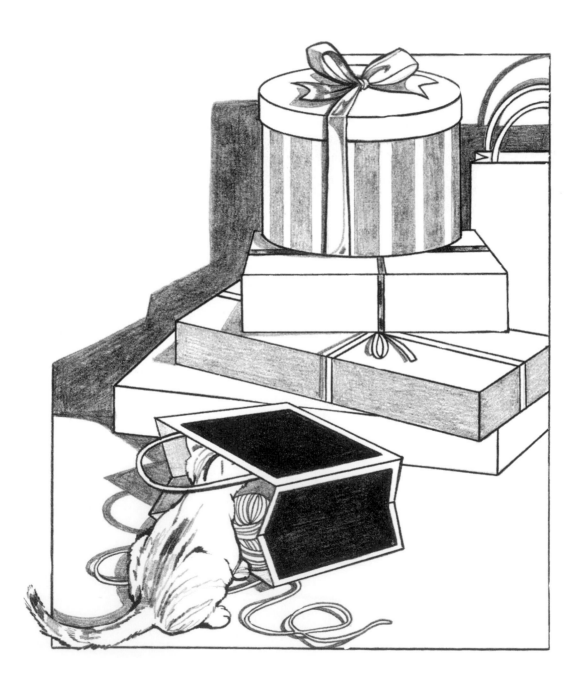

Get to know which manufacturers (or designers if you are lucky) consistently produce clothes that are cut well for you. With practice, you will be able to buy some clothes without even trying them on.

Shopping can be fun even if you don't have much time for it. Color makes it easier, faster, and more rewarding, since you know that whatever you buy in your colors will look great.

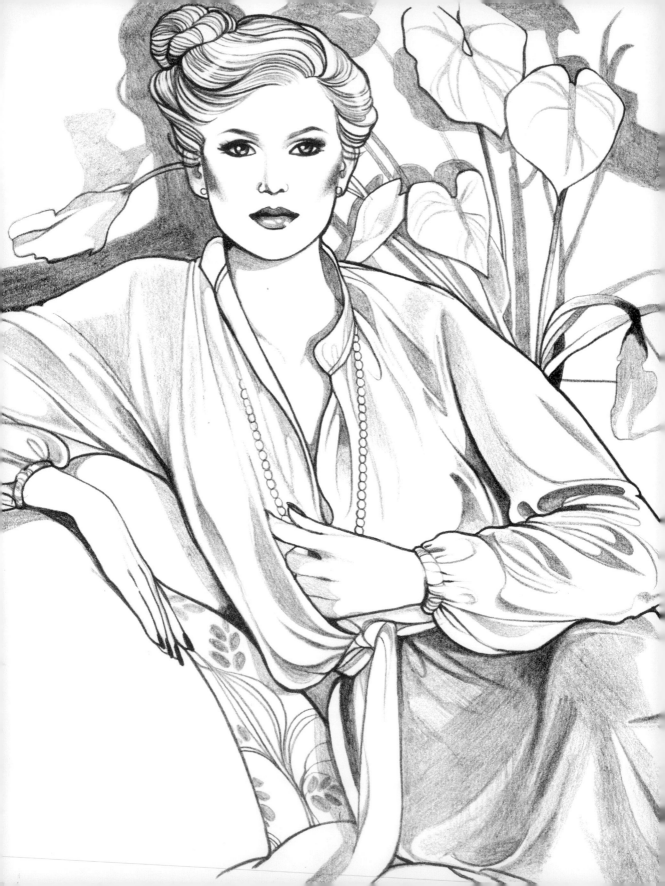

14

LET YOURSELF GLOW

NOW THAT COLOR HAS CHANGED YOUR OUTER IMAGE, USE IT TO change your self-image as well.

We have all seen the woman who, despite attractive features, perfect makeup, and immaculate grooming, radiates nothing. She looks good on the outside, but on the inside she feels like nobody, and that is the image she projects to others.

As you wear your colors, you can internalize the good looks and the compliments into good feelings, so that you not only look your best, but feel beautiful as a person—and that's the ultimate winning combination. The special magic of color is that your new image is authentically you, based not on fakery or "beauty tricks" but on flattery of the real you. You are not hiding what you don't like about yourself; you are revealing the best of yourself.

Let's summarize the steps you take to find your natural beauty and put your colors to work for you.

1. Take the color test to determine your season.

2. Study and understand your colors. "Shop" with your swatches and get to know your color "personality."

3. Start wearing your colors, beginning with what you have.

4. Start wearing the right makeup colors. Be particular about the shades. Correct makeup does make a difference and you need only one set.

5. Attend to your hair, in both color and style. Get rid of the wrong color as soon as possible. It really detracts.

6. Check out your closet and list the things you need, keeping the list with your swatches. Buy new clothes in your colors only. Always shop with your swatches. Your eye cannot retain color by memory and there are subtle differences in some shades.

7. As you shop, give thought to your type and the styles and accessories that most suit you. Watch for compliments as the signal you are on the right track.

8. Begin to build a wardrobe around basics.

Now, let yourself glow. The real fun comes as you develop your own sense of style, the look that says, "I am me." Style is not fashion. Style is the positive expression of your individuality, of both your inner and your outer personality.

Your colors alone do not give you style, but they help. It takes time and effort on your part to implement your new look and explore your clothing personality. But even if you don't develop a flair for dressing, you will achieve a statement of style and a put-together look from the dynamics of your palette alone.

As you wear your colors, you will find that you grow into your season and people begin to associate your colors with you, even in the gifts they choose for you. And you can use your colors to develop a style that can be expressed in every aspect of your life. Your home or office decor, the flowers you choose, your stationery, linens, china, even your wallet, umbrella, and car become a reflection of your own style and personality.

In your home, you can use your swatches to plan a color scheme. If you live with someone whose season is different from yours, mix the two by putting together compatible colors from both. Usually it's best to stick to two colors in a room decor and then tie them together with a neutral or pale version of one of the two colors. For example, you might mix Winter's yellow with Spring's light orange on a rug of neutral ivory or pale yellow. Because yellow and orange are warm, use Spring's warm palette to add a print or a small touch of an accent color. Your palette is an invaluable aid to decorating your home. It's rewarding—and flattering—to live in your colors, and be in harmony with your environment.

Develop your own ideas as you explore other ways to express your personality through your season. Here are some suggestions.

The Winter woman might choose flowers that are bold or formal—perhaps carnations or long-stemmed roses in colors from her palette. Summer's flowers would be softer—roses, gardenias, violets. Autumn might choose mums, zinnias, poppies, and large daisies, while Spring's flowers could be daisies, daffodils,

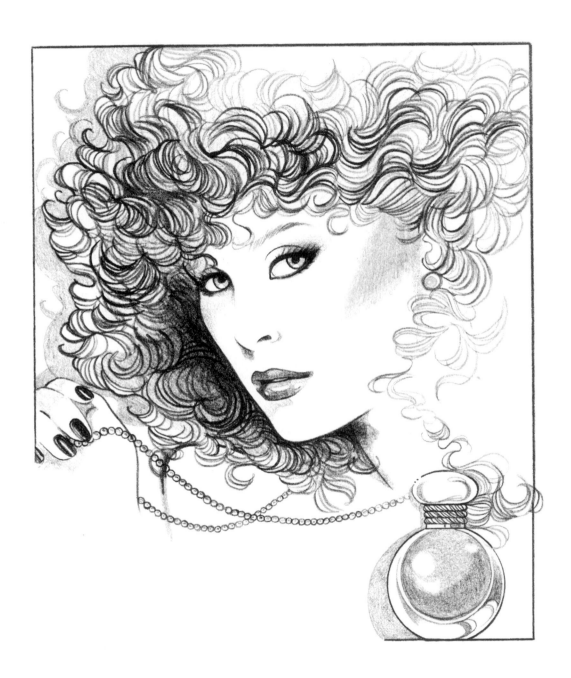

tulips, lilies of the valley, or baby rosebuds. Both the color and the "feeling" of the flowers in your home can reflect your personality.

Stationery for the cool Winter woman should be sophisticated, with perhaps a modern silver monogram. For Summer, the classic, traditional type with a script monogram is best. Autumn would choose rough paper with a heavy gold monogram, whereas Spring is most likely to be herself in delicate paper with a small, crisp monogram in gold.

Even your perfume personality can emerge from your season. While Winter is good in exotic, spicy scents, Summer is more the floral type. Autumn is best in woodsy or fruity fragrances and Spring in light, fresh, sweet smells from flowers or fruits.

Do you see how your palette can permeate your entire life style and even help you develop your identity?

So you are really not at the end of a book, but rather at the beginning of a whole new look, perhaps a new life. Color is not static. It is vital and dynamic. The real rewards are still in your future. You can color yourself beautiful in the truest sense of the word, with the glow—the beauty—that comes from total harmony and satisfaction with yourself.

Index

Color Me Beautiful

If you would like to purchase a set of fabric swatches in your season's colors plus an attractive carrying case, or want information on Carole Jackson™ cosmetics and other seasonalized products, call:

U.S. 800-533-5503
In Virginia: 800-572-2335
In Canada: 1-800-633-1010

or, write to the following address:
Carole Jackson
P.O. Box 3241
Falls Church, VA 22043

Color Me Beautiful

If you would like the names of the Color Me Beautiful consultants nearest you, or information on how to become a Consultant, call:

U.S. 800-533-5503
In Virginia: 800-572-2335
In Canada: 1-800-633-1010

or, write to the following address:
Carole Jackson
P.O. Box 3241
Falls Church, VA 22043